A MINNESOTA DOCTOR'S
HOME REMEDIES
FOR COMMON AND UNCOMMON
AILMENTS

Third Edition

Also by Dr. Eichenlaub

A MINNESOTA DOCTOR'S GUIDE TO WEIGHT REDUCTION
AND CONTROL

A MINNESOTA DOCTOR'S

HOME REMEDIES

FOR COMMON AND UNCOMMON

AILMENTS

THIRD EDITION

John E. Eichenlaub, M.D.

PRENTICE-HALL, INC.   Englewood Cliffs, N.J.

Prentice-Hall International, Inc., *London*
Prentice-Hall of Australia, Pty. Ltd., *Sydney*
Prentice-Hall of Canada, Ltd., *Toronto*
Prentice-Hall of India Private Ltd., *New Delhi*
Prentice-Hall of Japan, Inc., *Tokyo*
Prentice-Hall of South Asia Pte. Ltd., *Singapore*
Whitehall Books, Ltd., *Wellington, New Zealand*

©1981 by

John E. Eichenlaub, M.D.

This book is a reference work based on research by the author. The opinions expressed herein are not necessarily those of or endorsed by the publisher. The directions stated in this book are in no way to be considered as a substitute for consultation with a duly licensed doctor.

Library of Congress Cataloging in Publication Data

Eichenlaub, John E
  A Minnesota doctor's home remedies for common and uncommon ailments.

  Includes index.
  1. Medicine, Popular. I. Title.
RC81.E33   1980   616'.024   80-27588
ISBN 0-13-584532-7

Printed in the United States of America

What This Book of Home Remedies Can Do for You

Very few people can go to a doctor for every misery, hurt or disorder. They have to weigh their difficulties against the time and money a physician's care may consume. Unless they have considerable distress, they often shrug off their complaints as burdens to be borne, and carry on as well as they can.

If that is what you sometimes have to do, the home remedies and other measures you find in this book will help you greatly. You can cure or relieve many ailments right in your own home, often without spending a dime for medicines or doctor care, or a minute waiting in a doctor's office. You can perk yourself up and boost your resistance to disease with simple, inexpensive home tonics. You can take definite countermeasures and maintain informed alertness against serious disease and deterioration. This book gives you exact directions for hundreds of simple home remedies, tonics, and counteractants with which to meet or avoid about 200 mild and serious ailments. It solves the recurring dilemma of physician's care *vs.* stoical neglect by giving a third and often perfectly proper choice: well-managed, effective, convenient home measures.

Minnesota as home care center. An almost unique situation makes the Gopher State teem with tried and true home remedies. Although the isolation of old-time logging camps and wood-ringed farms has largely given way to modern progress, the hardy self-reliance of former days lives on. The people of this area usually go to the medicine chest instead of the nearest doctor when they get a sniffle or an ache. They can draw from all the traditions of Northern Europe as well as the scientific guidance of the medical centers at Rochester and Minneapolis. They have thousands of good doctors who are willing to correct and supplement home care instead of fighting it. No wonder Minnesotans get topnotch home care!

Another Scandinavian tradition is health promotion. No people in the world spend more effort building strength and vigor. When you think of Sweden, you think of calisthenics and gymnastic teams. Also, the thought of Finland brings the picture of steam-reddened bodies plunging into icy lakes for the sake of extra verve and vigor—a procedure that takes a world

1

of courage, and could never have been discovered without true dedication to the pursuit of health. Constant awareness of health problems is part of this tradition: our University's cancer detection clinic has a long waiting list; our heart hospital has a large department devoted to preventive care; our School of Public Health includes a world-famous center for studying the bodily processes and the strains of ordinary life. Home remedies in Minnesota go beyond care for common ailments to energy-building, zest-restoring tonics unknown in many other areas and to procedures aimed at finding or preventing deadly ills.

You and your family need home remedies. I am sure that all of you suffer some of the illnesses and disorders considered in this book. Muscle and join paints, indigestion, constipation, sex organ irritations, sluggish circulation, etc.—few families escape all of these common disorders for even a month at a time. How many hours of misery could sound home treatment have saved you in the past year? How much lost time and patent medicine money? Perhaps you have even had expensive and uncomfortable doctor's care which proper home measures could have made unnecessary! You can take eight different steps to cure yourself of muscular backache and to keep it from troubling you again. You can rid yourself of corns and callouses forever with three simple measures. You can choose from 16 completely different approaches to joint misery, ranging from hormone-stimulating aspirin doses and warm flannel application to special massage, paraffin baths, and sleep-aiding braces. You can solve your constipation problem for good with the step-by-step home method outlined in Chapter 4. If rectal troubles have plagued you, learn how to distinguish hemorrhoids from splits or fissures and what curative measures you can take against each of these common miseries. Don't let aftermaths of motherhood like cystocoel and rectocoel build their discomforts through the years either: a slight change in the position you assume for emptying your bowel might save you the misery and expense of a later operation. And if you have had sex complaints—whether male or female—Chapter 7 provides a broad assortment of remedies you can apply in the privacy of your own home. Other chapters deal with sinus trouble, stuffy noses, nasal crusts. These and other nose and throat discomforts yield to measures you can readily adopt. Home remedies give quick relief for many skin troubles, too, including conditions like eczema and psoriasis, for which no amount of prescription care brings permanent and lasting cure.

Even if you presently have none of these miseries or the dozens of others treated in the pages of this book, the chances are that you will have several occasions to use its helpful guidance during the next year. How many people live 12 months without a cold, without a scrape, bruise, or burn, without a boil or skin eruption? You can apply the specific, concrete directions that this book offers to all of these and to many other common ailments. If you get a headache, for instance, you will find separate sections with exact treatment suggestions, for each of the seven common varieties of head pain. From itching scalp to ingrown toenail, you'll find exact, complete directions for handling home care of over 200 different disorders.

The world's most practical treatments! Most of the home remedies in this book call for substances and ingredients you can find in any household—hot and cold water, salt, baking soda, paraffin, and vinegar, for instance. Many of the others depend on standard medicine chest items like nose drops, rubbing alcohol, and petroleum jelly. You can buy almost all of the other materials needed without a prescription in your drugstore or supermarket. In a few instances, when the materials available without prescription are in a less convenient form (e.g., non-prescription stomach-soothing suppositories vs. prescription pills) or are less economical (e.g., swallowed doses of relatively expensive ephedrine nose drops), the prescription equivalent has been included, too. You may want to ask your doctor to prescribe these remedies for your medicine chest when you next visit his office.

Tone up for vigorous living! Maybe it's the lure of 11,000 lovely lakes and 19 million acres of timberland, or maybe it's plain distaste for feeling old, but Minnesotans have more ways of toning up themselves than any other group I know. Several of their favorite techniques, detailed in Chapter 14, measurably increase your energy and vigor. Dr. Keys of Minnesota's Laboratory of Physiological Hygiene has been a front runner in investigations of health-improving foods, too. The concrete, three-step dietary program (described in Chapter 16) for staving off hardened arteries and the other ravages once thought to be an inevitable part of old age is largely an outgrowth of his and other studies done right in this state. One thing I'll guarantee: you will definitely feel new zest and vigor through the fatigue-dispelling exercises, the stimulating home tonic methods and the nerve-soothing tranquilizing techniques that this book spells out. Procedures like the cold friction bath, the sheet bath, and the specially conducted rest period can lighten the burden of your daily life from this moment forth.

Counteract serious ailments and disorders. You have one advantage that even your doctor does not enjoy in fighting off illness: you can take action day by day to boost your resistance, and to ward off or detect the bare beginnings of disease. Action *right now* can cut your chance of suffering such conditions as the common cold, ulcers, skin infection, hardened arteries, coronary heart attacks, and even cancer. Learn to avoid these and many other health hazards with simple home measures! An ounce of prevention is worth more than a pound of cure. You can head off many plagues that no doctor on earth can stop once they have a grip on you. Corrective measures you can take right in your own home will add extra, youthful, vigorous, misery-free years to your lifespan. You'll find exact techniques outlined in full detail throughout this book.

Use doctor's care more effectively than ever before, too. You can make your doctor's care much more effective with home techniques, even when home remedies will not suffice. Learn to spot the illnesses and complications for which very prompt medical care is cheaper and better. Learn actual home techniques for identifying possibly serious health problems early, when your doctor's care will do you the most good. Learn how to make procedures like gall bladder surgery and the care of heart attacks much easier on you and much more effective. The measures advised in this book are realistic: they do not send you to your doctor for every sniffle. But they do reveal many ways in which you can get more help from your doctor without extra medical expense.

Home remedies, tonics and counteractants can help YOU. Make no mistake: a great many of the miseries and discomforts you have suffered will yield to home remedies. *You* can fight off illness and disease without undue expense or inconvenience. *You* can make yourself feel younger, more vigorous, and more cheerful by using home tonics. *You* can counteract threats of serious disease and deterioration with day-by-day home measures. Countless Minnesotans have tried the how-to techniques outlined in this book over a period of many years. Some of the country's finest doctors have helped weed out the old wives' tales from the genuine, useful remedies and have added their own wisdom to the fine distillate of Northern Europe's finest healing traditions. The results are all here, in this book. Won't you put its hundreds of practical remedies and tonics to work for you today?

John E. Eichenlaub, M.D.

Why This Third Edition?

When someone asked Isaac Newton how he achieved his great scientific discoveries, such as the law of gravity, he said: "By standing on the shoulders of giants."

This third edition came into being in much the same way. Literally thousands of people have added impetus, either knowingly or unknowingly, until the book simply had to burst forth.

First there was YOU, the readers of prior editions, whose feedback through letters, live-audience contact and personal consultation has pointed up many ways in which the book could be made more useful and interesting. The new chapter on weight control and the section dealing with specific problems of people in their sixties and seventies fit in this category.

Second, a horde of health workers and dedicated research personnel have brought countless new ideas into the field of home care. Yesterday's facts in this area often prove to be today's outmoded beliefs. Although the advances that make the headlines deal with mortal illnesses and highly technical procedures, progress affects home care, too. The new material on low blood sugar, choking, and food allergy are examples. Many of the facts reported in this edition weren't known at the time of the prior editions.

Third, the marvelous process of democracy has proved itself again, and the freedom and welfare of YOU, the people, has won out over certain special interests. About fifteen years ago in a legislative hearing here in Minnesota, the head of the state pharmacy association testified that his organization's aim was to make *every* effective remedy "prescription only." And for many years that philosophy carried great weight with the federal Food and Drug Administration, which sharply limited the products you could buy without a prescription and the places you could buy them. But the voice of the consumer seems to have penetrated even the FDA's marble halls, because in the past few years that agency has released a whole host of safe, effective remedies. Now you can get the benefit of home products which dramatically help allergy, skin rash, superficial infections, common colds and dozens of other conditions for which almost all of the most effective medications were previously "prescription only." All of these products have been thoroughly tested and proved for safety and effectiveness, and do not involve the hazards that you may think of in connection with artificial chemicals and strong drugs. And I've included in this book those in which I have complete confidence, such as bacitracin (on which my father did much of the original research) and proper-strength cortisone ointments, selected antihistamines, improved cold remedies and new spasm-soothers to aid digestion.

Finally, let me once again give credit to the marvelous reception YOU the reader have given to the previous editions of this book. Simply knowing that literally millions of you have valued my advice and accepted my judgment has been a constant source of satisfaction and a real spur to continued effort in bringing this new and even more useful material into print. Thank you once more for your confidence and your support.

John E. Eichenlaub, M.D.

ACKNOWLEDGMENT

My thanks to my wife Pat, who not only spurred my creative urges and smoothed the pathway of life to facilitate my own efforts but also took over many of the chores connected with making this edition a reality. Also to Janet Sjoselius, who translated my illegible scrawls into meaningful typescript.

Contents

Muscular Backache (19). Hot showers with Figure 8 movement. Shower massage. Aspirin. Extra sleep support. Paraffin baths. Massage. Conquer a tendency toward backache. **Muscular Miseries, Cramps, and Charley Horses (22).** Relieve aching muscles. Neck and shoulder-arm pain. Thoracic outlet syndrome. Muscle cramps. Charley horses. **Foot Troubles (27).** Trim corns and callouses. Relieve pressure to rid yourself of corns and callouses. Felt pads. Relief from blisters. Relief for painful arches. Adolescent arch strain. Tricks for taping. Tape for arch strain. Long-range help with arch troubles. Jogger's foot. Bunions. Ingrown toenail. Thickened and deformed nails.

Does Hypoglycemia Cause Any Problems for You? (34). A self-testing technique for hypoglycemia. Subtle forms of hypoglycemia. Hypoglycemia diet. Severe forms of hypoglycemia. **Food Allergy (39).** How to tell if you have a food allergy. Major detection methods. Minor detection methods. Doctors and food allergy. **The Gist of This Chapter (46).**

Joint Pains (47). Red, swollen joints. The hormone-stimulating aspirin dose. Red joints in children. Warm flannel. Diet. Bodily rest. Rest for sore joints. Motion-preserving exercises. Supported or flotation exercises. Cripple-cutting braces. Subsiding or smoldering joint trouble. Sore, stiff fingers. Jogger's knee. Aching arms, hips, or knees. Perpetual stiff neck. Stiff elbows, wrists, ankles, and toes. Tennis elbow. Diffuse joint trouble. Home whirlpool equipment. Hip, knee, and joint strain. Growing pains. **Neuritis, Bursitis, and Inflamed Leader Guides (56).** Neuritis and neuralgia. Bursitis. Leader guide inflammation.

borne ride. **Heart and Artery Trouble (225).** Heart complaints don't mean heart trouble even half the time. Even real heart failure can be stopped before it starts. Twinges of heart misery give valuable warning. Sluggish heart action. Rheumatic fever. **Innocent Chest Pains (227).** Gas pains. **Hardening of the Arteries (228).** A controllable disease. Why cholesterol forms scales within artery walls. Attacks on the artery-hardening mechanism. The fat you eat determines the cholesterol in your blood. Keep down the amount of harmful fat. Use liquid cooking oils. Keep down the total fuel value of foods. An artery-preserving diet. Even easy artery-sparing diets may soon be unnecessary. **Avoid Coronary Heart Trouble (232).** Open coronary arteries with muscular activity. Aspirin. Wholesome outlets for pent-up emotion. Meet some resentments specifically. **Keep Your Blood Pressure Down (237).** Dodging excess salt. Self-assertion. Getting reassurance. Doctoring for blood pressure.

17. HOW TO MEET AND CONQUER TUMOR THREATS ... 239

Avoid many cancers. Irritation spurs cancerous growth. **Cancer-Spurring Irritations (240).** Cancer-causing ultraviolet rays. Protect your lungs against dangerous fumes and irritants. What about tobacco? **How to Quit Smoking (241).** Breathing exercises really work. Cleansing intimate body parts. **Help Your Doctor to Fight Cancer-Spurring Irritation (243).** Cancer-spurring states at the mouth of the womb. Your dentist can help you dodge cancer. **Innocent Growths and Cancer Vanguards (244).** Warts. Ganglion. Skin tags. **Spot Cancer Vanguards Yourself (245).** Heaped-up skin cells. White patches. Moles. **Your Doctor Can Help Find and Remove Tumor Threats (246).** Doctors find cancer vanguards you'd never see. Doctors cure many cancers completely. A sore or spot that does not heal. A lump, bunch, or bulge. Unusual bleeding. Unusual flux or discharge. Lasting stomach trouble. Change in bowel habits. Change in voice or altered cough.

18. HOW TO RELIEVE WEIGHT-RELATED STRAINS ON YOUR SYSTEM 250

When Weight Loss Is Urgent (250). Long-term help with weight control. The mental and emotional side of weight con-

trol. **Solve Your Weight Problem with Fitting Substitutions**
(253). Substitute protein and fiber for starch and fat. Substitute
heightened flavor and better seasoning for richness. Substitute
eye appeal for volume. Substitute solids for liquids. Substitute
sometime—almost anything—for your Weight Waterloos.
Substitute a low-cal drink for beer or booze. **Weight Control**
Summary (256). Quick Weight Loss Diet (257). Foods to
Choose for Long-Range Weight Control (258).

A MINNESOTA DOCTOR'S
HOME REMEDIES
FOR COMMON AND UNCOMMON
AILMENTS

Third Edition

1

New Home Remedies for Muscular Backache, Muscle Miseries and Foot Troubles

There's one time when our sturdy Minnesotans are not too proud of their strength and hardihood: when those bulging muscles begin to hurt. With almost forty inches of snow to shovel each year, muscular backaches sometimes seem to be the Gopher State's pet affliction. Even the happy exertions of a canoe trip through wilderness or a long hike through the color riot of the autumn forest sometimes impose later punishment in the form of stiff leg muscles or aching feet. Our hardy folk have learned to get to work on those discomforts right away with home measures, which usually bring quick relief.

HOME MEASURES AGAINST MUSCULAR BACKACHE

You can take effective steps right in your own home to relieve backache and keep it from troubling you further. The equipment you need costs very little, but will often give you complete relief. Here are specific directions:

Hot showers with Figure 8 movement. When your back begins to hurt after a session of difficult lifting and bending, you should start toward relief right away. A hot shower in the proper position will work wonders. Stand with both knees slightly bent and both hands on your thighs just above the knee. Rest a good bit of your weight on your arms to relieve your tired back of the burden. Drape a towel over your back, being sure to cover the affected area. Let a needle spray of hot water play through the towel on the sore area. Now pretend that you are drawing tiny figure 8's in the air with the lower end of your spine. Raise and push back one hip slightly, raise and push back the other hip, return to normal position, lower and tuck in one hip, lower and tuck in the other. Repeat slowly for about ten minutes.

Your youngsters can use this same approach to avoid backache and stiffness after contact sports. I've actually seen several of the University of Minnesota's Golden Golpher football teams going through this routine on the trainer's orders after a tough game or a trying workout. When your youngsters get into slam-bang athletics, show them this passage and let them give special showers a try.

Shower massage. Special shower heads which give alternating pulses of water under high pressure have added a new dimension to home care of muscular disorders. I have one made by Water-Pik in my own bathroom, and find it a real boon for soothing stiff or aching muscles after exercising and for relieving my morning stiffness (which I blame on residuals of rheumatism, not caring to admit that it might simply be an affliction of age). The pulses can be set for different rhythm and intensity, and the water can either be allowed to strike your skin directly or transmitted through a towel. Using a towel intensifies the effect of the heat by keeping hot water in contact with the entire area and does not interfere with the massage, but the simpler direct impact method works well for most minor discomforts. Start with rapid, low intensity massage, moving your body so that the stream impact moves along the sore muscles either up and down (on the back) or up along a stiff arm or leg. After a minute or two, adjust the shower head to give stronger, less frequent pulses and repeat the movement. Other shower massage devices are available, some with flexible extension tubes which allow easier treatment of such areas as the calves and feet. Cost is moderate, anyone can do the installation with an ordinary monkey wrench, and this kind of massage gives a lot of relief.

Aspirin. If the backache develops in spite of this maneuver, take aspirin after each meal and at bedtime for at least two days, two tablets at a dose if you weigh 150 pounds or less, three if you weigh more than 150. Continue half doses after pain subsides as long as you have any back discomfort whatever. Youngsters below age twelve usually heal faster without aspirin than with it, probably because they go back to full activity as soon as you relieve their discomfort.

Extra sleep support. You will get a great deal of relief from sleeping on a firm bed. Sag-free sleeping lets your weight stretch tight muscles when sleep relaxes them, and definitely helps you to get well. A piece of one-inch plywood underneath a cotton mattress prevents sag. Put this arrangement on top of box or coil springs for firm but yielding support. Or use an extra-firm orthopedic type foam rubber or innerspring mattress.

Paraffin baths. Paraffin gives at least as much benefit as expensive tissue-heating machine treatments which many patients take for back trouble. Paraffin baths are safe and inexpensive. You can learn the technique in five minutes and re-use the same materials for weeks or months. Here are the details:

Get the following materials together:
1-2 lbs. paraffin, of the type sold in grocery and drug stores for sealing preserves.
Mineral oil.
Double boiler.
Dry towels.
Paint brush, with rubber-set bristles.

Melt the paraffin in the double boiler. Add 2 tablespoonfuls of mineral oil for each pound of paraffin. Let the mixture cool until a definite scum forms on the top. Break the scum and test further by putting in a half-inch square of paraffin, which should not melt when the temperature is right. Oil or shave the back if it is very hairy. Have a member of your family paint your back with the paraffin. After the first layer is firm, paint on another. Continue until paraffin is about ¼ inch thick. Cover with a dry towel to hold the heat. After thirty to forty-five minutes, remove the towel and peel off the paraffin-oil mixture. You will find that it comes off very easily. Save it, and use the same mixture over and over again. Add further oil to make later applications cooler, or add pure paraffin to make peeling easier if you will tolerate slightly higher temperatures.

After you get accustomed to the heat and the procedure, you may want to use pure paraffin instead of paraffin-oil mixture. Pure paraffin gives maximum heat and maximum benefit.

Massage. You can get a great deal of relief from backache with properly done massage. This treatment is especially effective if it follows immediately after a paraffin bath. Here's the technique:

Strip and lie on your abdomen on a comfortable but firm surface. Get your helper to start with rhythmic top-to-bottom strokes along the muscle masses beside the spine. He can lubricate the skin with mineral oil or with liniment made from one part methyl salicylate (oil of wintergreen) and two parts camphor and soap liniment. After about five minutes of gentle stroking, when the tight back muscles begin to loosen up and relax somewhat, a kneading type of massage may prove helpful. This begins at the upper back. Your helper presses his fingers firmly (but not uncomfortably) into the muscle mass beside the spine. Continuing pressure, he moves them up and down as far as the elasticity of the skin permits. Then he slides the fingers down about one inch and repeats the kneading motion. He continues in this fashion down the length of the spine, and repeats the procedure for about five minutes. He should then go back to gentle stroking and taper the pressure and rhythm to a soothing conclusion for the massage. If you used mineral oil for lubrication, clean it off with rubbing alcohol. If you use the liniment, you will find that it soaks in.

How to conquer a tendency toward backache. You can prevent recurrence of most muscular backaches with simple home exercises. The muscles of your abdomen work through the leverage of your rib cage and pelvis to brace your back. The heavy muscles near the spine also do their part. Extra strength in these muscle groups makes a natural girdle which supports your spine from every angle, thus preventing most muscular backache and many more serious back injuries.

After a bout with backache, wait until your back is fairly comfortable, then strengthen your back-bracing muscles with these exercises, best done as you are getting up in the morning:

1. Relieve pressure on nerves at the spinal cord exits with a simple stretching exercise. Before you get out of bed, draw both knees up to your chest or even into your armpits, drawing the low back to its maximum forward-arching position. Pull firmly enough to feel stretch in the back muscles three or four times.

2. Strengthen the muscles at the sides of your spinal column by standing erect and raising one leg straight out to the side as far as it will go. Repeat thirty times on each side.

3. Strengthen abdominal muscles with leg straightening. Lie on your back with your knees drawn up and your hands beside your hips. Slowly straighten your legs, keeping your feet about six inches above the floor. If the strain on the abdominal muscles becomes too great, do not try to straighten your legs all the way at first. When you have straightened them as far as is comfortable, slowly fold them again. Repeat five times.

4. For further abdominal strengthening, spread your arms straight to the sides while lying on your back. Stretch out your legs with your feet about twelve inches apart. Slowly lift your right leg until it is perpendicular, and bring your foot across to touch the floor high up beside your left hip. Return your right leg by reversing the motions, and follow the same pattern with your left leg. Repeat five times.

For best results, you should do these exercises daily for the rest of your life. Most people do them religiously until they have been free of pain for a few months, then slack off. Unfortunately the cure only lasts as long as the effort, and you are quite likely to have more trouble whenever you stop taking the exercises.

HOME MEASURES FOR MUSCULAR MISERIES, CRAMPS, AND CHARLEY HORSES

When the earlier editions of this book came out, my muscular misery patients usually came to the office in their overalls. Good solid folks who had to wrestle with crates of bales of hay, poor housewives who lugged wet wash because they couldn't afford a clothes dryer, husky laborers who eked out a living at the end of a shovel. A few of those folks still trickle in, in spite of the way workman's compensation has forced most bosses to provide hydraulic lifts. But the far more typical muscle strain victim nowadays tells a story of stress and strain while jogging or misery following his early efforts to "get back in shape." Not that I'm against the exercise craze—on balance I'm sure that active people stay healthier and live longer without heart attacks or other serious disease. But there's no doubt that the result has made this chapter important to almost everyone: the poor because they still *have to* strain those muscles and the not-so-poor because they nowadays *choose to* do so.

How to relieve aching muscles. At the first sign of muscular aching after any unusual work or muscle strain, start a three-pronged attack on muscle miseries:

Take aspirin. Start with two tablets after each meal and at bedtime if you weigh less than 150 pounds, three tablets at a dose if you weigh 150 pounds or more. Continue for at least two days, whether you think you need it or not. Then take half doses until the misery is completely gone.

Apply heat. A tub bath with moderately hot water, between 98 and 108 degrees, may be very helpful for general aching. If only one or two muscles are sore, you may get relief with hot towels, folded until six to eight layers thick, dipped in water at about 112 degrees, and covered with a dry towel to help hold the heat. Hot towels are more helpful if they are applied somewhat toward the heart from the sore area as well as directly over it: treat a sore forearm with hot towels wrapped nearly to the shoulder, for instance.

Improve blood drainage. A very substantial portion of muscular aching is due to accumulated chemical wastes. You can relieve this condition with circulation-aiding massage and downhill drainage. The aching extremity should be arranged on pillows so that it is several inches above the level of your chest. Slow massage is very helpful, using limp fingers, rhythmic strokes and mineral oil for lubrication. Each stroke of the massage should start at the most distant point from the heart and run up the affected extremity. After ten minutes or so of gentle stroking, a somewhat deeper pressure with the palm of the hand often helps, milking body juices from the sore area toward the heart. Five minutes or so of such milking, followed by a gradual taper to very gentle massage again, gives a great deal of relief and definitely speeds healing. Clean off the mineral oil with rubbing alcohol. Repeat the procedure once or twice a day until the aching subsides.

Neck and shoulder-arm pain. Years ago at Minnesota's Mayo Clinic one of my doctor friends found his office filled with a steady succession of hard-working farm and laboring people with neck and shoulder-arm pain. He knew that this pain often stemmed from one of life's great vicious circles: muscular discomfort leading to muscle spasm which in turn pinches nerves and leads to further discomfort. Time after time, my friend relieved victims of persistent or recurrent miseries by stretching over-tight muscles. The key step, he found, was stretching the muscles around the spinal column in the neck and upper back. At first, he did this with a special leather head halter and a complicated arrangement of pulleys and weights. As the years went by, however, my friend saw that many poor workers had to stay away from their homes for weeks at a time and many good Minnesota farmers had to trek miles several times each week to take full advantage of this treatment. His new device uses a water bag for weight and attaches to the top of a door. You can buy it at any orthopedic supply store.

You can often get a great deal of help with any kind of muscular or arthritic discomfort in the neck, upper back, or shoulder and arm with home-fashioned means of neck stretching. If you can't afford to buy a head sling from the nearest surgical supply house, you can make one out of table felt from any dry goods store. Start with a double thickness two inches wide and two yards long. Sew the ends together solidly to make a single loop. Put your head through the middle of this loop and hold the ends of it with one hand in the vicinity of each shoulder. Twist the ends you have in your hands half a turn, so that the loop crosses itself at each side of your neck. Raise the two ends up above your head, keeping the center portion of the loop tucked under your chin in the front and beneath the curve of your head in the back. At the point where the strips cross above your ears, pin with two safety pins. Adjust so that the head sling will slip on and off easily and so that the side loops are approximately equal in length. Replace the pins with firm stitching if you wish.

Whether you buy or make your head sling, you will need to suspend a sturdy wooden coat hanger directly over your head. A hook screwed into a door frame or other support works very well to hold the coat hanger. After adjusting the sling at your chin and the nape of your neck, put the side loops or traction traps of the sling across the coat hanger arms. Bend your knees slightly so that your body weight produces steady muscle-stretching action all along the upper spine. Adjust the sling so that your head remains upright instead of tipping backward during the stretch, and settle down for a steady five to ten minute spasm soothing session. Some of my Minnesota angler patients put a spring type fish-scale between the coat hanger and the supporting hook or eyelet to help them determine how much to bend their knees. Ten to 15 pounds is the limit with recent or extreme neck pain. Victims of smoldering, long-lasting miseries sometimes must work gradually up to 50 pounds.

Thoracic outlet syndrome. One special form of neck and shoulder-arm pain occurs quite frequently and causes a great deal of misery. This stems from pressure on nerves as they pass through a narrow canal just above the first rib. This canal also contains the main artery which leads to the arm, and anything that causes pressure on the nerves will also cut off flow in the artery under some circumstances. This permits a simple home test for a narrowed thoracic outlet canal, which you can do in a few seconds. Simply locate the pulse in your wrist and be sure that you can feel it easily. Then raise your arm straight out to the side from your body and bend your elbow so that the forearm points straight forward. If you have a narrow thoracic outlet canal, you will find that your pulse is either very weak or totally undetectable when your arm is in this position.

Under these circumstances, three measures usually prove worthwhile:

1. Avoid any work above your head. Not only will your arm become numb from blood vessel pressure if you try to do such a job as painting the ceiling or putting up acoustic tile, but the nerve irritation that occurs at the same time that the circulation is impaired may cause pain and misery that might go on for months.

2. Avoid using the affected hand as a pillow when you sleep. Some of my patients have continued to have shoulder-arm pain until they made a tether to wear at night—an old belt around the chest, a felt cuff for the arm, and a length of cord to connect the two with enough slack for comfort and not enough to allow the arm to be raised more than a few inches.

3. If shoulder-arm pain develops, put hot compresses on the arm where the pressure occurs, above the collarbone at the base of the neck, rather than where you feel the discomfort. Twenty minutes three or four times a day often gives considerable relief.

Muscle cramps. Gentle kneading, preferably through several layers of warm, wet towel or with the part immersed in warm water, gives quick relief from ordinary muscle cramps. The towels or water should be lukewarm, not hot (about 98 degrees). Start kneading somewhat below the cramped muscle, keeping your fingers together and using their flat surfaces instead of their tips. Knead upward toward the trunk as if you were working oleomargarine in a plastic bag. Repeat several times with gradually deeper kneading. A warm flannel wrap helps to keep down later soreness.

If you get muscle cramps mainly from swimming or unusual exertion, you can usually control your tendency toward them by taking several simple precautions:

Extra salt. Exertion causes sweating. Sweat carries salt out of your body. Unless you take enough salt to replace what you lose, muscle fibers become irritable from the low salt level in tissue fluids around them. This muscle irritability is the cause of most cramps at work, in the swimming pools, and at sporting events. Big time football players dodge this problem by drinking a solution of half a teaspoonful of salt to each glass of water whenever they practice or play. You can use the same approach, or you can take heat fatigue type salt tablets if you prefer—one tablet for each extra glass of water you drink.

Vein flushing exercises. Leg cramps that come on after you have been standing a great deal usually are due to accumulation of chemical wastes in the muscles. Your leg veins do not flush chemical wastes out of your muscles very effectively when you are standing, especially if you have any varicose veins. The best way to keep from getting leg cramps is to take time out every two hours when you are on your feet to do this exercise: Take off your shoes and socks. Lie on your back with hips raised on a pillow or on the arm of an overstuffed davenport or chair. Put your feet high in the air, and jiggle them rapidly with the ankles and toes completely relaxed for a period of 30 seconds.

Bed cradles. Muscle cramps during the night often stop if you keep the weight of covers off your feet. Trim two ordinary cardboard cartons from the grocery store down to an upright rectangle of cardboard for the bottom of the bed, a bracing triangle at each side, and a steadying base to tuck under the mattress. Put these cardboard corners in place over the bottom sheet and underneath the other covers. If you find the extra comfort you obtain with supported bedclothing is worthwhile, you may want to buy a metal bed cradle from your druggist or surgical supply house.

Quinine. If night cramps persist in spite of support for bedclothing, take one quinine tablet (five grains) each day for ten days. This usually gives at least six months relief. Quinine is perfectly safe in this dosage unless you are pregnant or have disease of the arteries, in which case you should check with your doctor first. You should time dosage to avoid menstrual periods.

Charley horses. A Charley horse is a muscle cramp which is so severe that it wrenches some muscle fibers loose and causes bleeding into the muscle itself. The blood which leaks out between muscle fibers causes irritation and further muscle spasm.

Cold. Immediate first aid for a Charley horse aims at shrinking blood vessels to limit internal bleeding. An ice pack is the best measure, and should be available at athletic contests and other places where muscle strain is expected.

Heat. You can safely use heat after an hour or so in treating a Charley horse. Muscle tissue contains a special substance which makes blood vessels seal themselves off almost instantly, so that further seepage of the kind which makes bruises extend themselves does not occur. Hot towels or hot soaks give considerable relief.

Other measures. Contrast baths, as described under "Painful Arches" on page 29, help if soreness persists. Gentle kneading massage for ten minutes after heat treatment may help to speed healing, too.

HOME CARE FOR FOOT TROUBLES

Almost everyone suffers at times from corns and callouses, blisters, and ingrown toenails, aching arches, or tired feet. Foot miseries are big miseries. If your feet hurt, you hurt all over. If your feet are tired, you are tired all over. Here's what to do for immediate relief and for permanent, lifelong cure of most common foot troubles:

How to trim corns and callouses. You can trim your own corns and callouses safely, unless you have diabetes or disease of the arteries. Wash your feet thoroughly and soak them in warm water for twenty minutes. Soak a new single-edged razor blade in rubbing alcohol, and use the same disinfectant to clean the corn or callous and the nearby skin. Wash your hands. Trim from the edge of the corn or callous toward the center, your blade almost parallel to the skin. Quit if you draw blood. Check with your doctor if you can't trim what seems to be a callous without drawing blood: you may have a wart that needs special treatment.

Relieve pressure to rid yourself of corns and callouses. Pressure, not rubbing, actually causes most corns and callouses. You can actually rid yourself of corns and callouses by properly fitted shoes, possibly with some felt pads. Properly fitted shoes also reduce foot strain and take much of the ache out of sagging arches. In checking my own patients, I've found about one in five grossly misfitted. The only way to be sure your shoes are right for you is to double check the fit yourself. Here's how to do it:

1. Check length by feeling for the ball of your foot, not the end of your toes. Feel along the side of the shoe and locate the knob at the base of your big toe, which should be just at the sharpest-curving point on the inside edge of your shoe sole. Always check standing as well as sitting because your feet may spread half a size or more under the burden of your body weight. Fit the longer foot, if they are different.

2. Check width. Feel for fit across the front of your foot and your little toe, with at least part of your weight on the foot. Pressure, not rubbing, causes blisters, corns, and callouses. Be sure you have enough room for your little toe when your weight is on your foot.

3. Check the shoes for bight. When you roll your weight up on the front part of your foot at the beginning of each step, creases in the leather may pinch you. Spot this while you're still in the store, and have the salesman put in a bight block to prevent it.

4. See whether the heel fits snugly, or whether it slips up and down easily. If you can't get shoes that fit both the front and the back of your foot properly, fit the front of your foot and get the heel padded or taken in. Most good shoe stores will fit a butterfly-shaped felt pad into your heels at no extra charge, with one wing on each side and a narrow strip around the back. Or you can get a shoemaker to take in the heel or fit molded heel counters, either of which should cost about four dollars.

Felt pads. If perfectly fitted shoes still leave slight pressure or friction at certain spots on your foot or if bony prominences push out against the skin, padding may be the only answer. However, *the object of padding is to spread weight or pressure to other parts of the foot or other parts of the affected bone, not to cushion the sore spot itself.* A thin layer of table felt cemented to the side and top of your shoe to hold the outer edge of your foot away from the leather may help corns. Some patients find that a sleeve of felt about four inches wide around the foot from the ankle to the base of the toes takes the weight off of callouses at the front of the foot and holds the leather away from corns simultaneously. If your toes curl sharply or if the end of one or more foot bones carries an undue share of weight so that it pushes against the skin from inside, a special type of felt pad called a metatarsal bar may help. A metatarsal bar attaches to the inside of your sole near the front of your arch. It cures corns by shifting the position of the toes on the ends of the foot bones so that they stay straight instead of curling. It cures callouses by spreading the weight across all four small foot bones instead of letting too much of it rest on one or two bone ends. Many shoe and drug stores sell metatarsal bars in three thicknesses and several sizes. Try medium thickness first. Determine where to place them in your shoes by laying a lead pencil on its side and stepping on it barefooted. Try first with the pencil about one inch behind the front of your arch, at the same angle as the bases of your four smaller toes. Find the exact space and angle at which your toes curl the least and your feet feel most comfortable. Then glue the metatarsal bars to the corresponding spot in your shoes.

If you wear many different pairs of shoes, you may find it more practical to use a leather insole with metatarsal pads. You can usually obtain this device at an orthopedic appliance store. Separate leather pouches permit insertion of different thickness pads under the ends of each foot bone, allowing completely individualized support. The insoles can be moved from one pair of shoes to another in a jiffy, so you only need one pair. Cost is somewhat higher than the ordinary metatarsal bar—generally about $20.

Relief from blisters. If new shoes or unusual exertions give you blisters on the hands or feet, adhesive tape bracing usually gives prompt relief. Wash the blistered part thoroughly with soap and water. Let it dry. Cut several four-inch strips of inch-wide cloth adhesive tape. Apply the center of one strip to the blister with at least ¼ inch of its upper margin on normal skin and smooth the ends into contact with the skin. Apply other overlapping strips until the entire blister and a margin of normal skin is smoothly covered with tape. Leave this in place for five days, then remove. The dead surface layer of the blister usually hangs limp by this time. You can trim it off with scissors or let it dry.

If the blister bursts before you get a chance to apply tape, or if it is larger than half a dollar, you can wash the area thoroughly, trim off the blister's roof, and keep a bandage lined with Telfa or a mild antiseptic ointment in place over it for four or five days.

Relief for painful arches. You can get a lot of relief from arch discomfort with "contrast baths." Fill one bucket or basin with moderately hot water, another with moderately cold. Ideal temperatures are 105 degrees and 50 degrees, but these need not be exact. Soak the affected part in hot water for four minutes, in cold for one minute, then back into the hot. Alternate for about thirty minutes. Always begin and end with the hot soak.

Massage also helps painful feet, especially if it is done immediately after a contrast bath. The object of the massage is to milk strain-produced chemical wastes out of the feet and ankles, not to rub the sore ligaments and muscles. You should lie down with your legs comfortably arranged on two or more pillows. Dry the legs thoroughly and powder them well with talc. If you have a helper, ask him to make a collapsible ring by joining the tips of his thumbs and forefingers. Starting at the base of the toes, he should draw this finger-thumb ring up the length of the foot and lower leg, milking blood and tissue fluid toward the heart. Repeat rhythmically with gradually increasing pressure for five to ten minutes, tapering off to gentle pressure before ending the massage. If you have no one to help you, you can lie on your back with one or two pillows under your hips and your legs drawn up. In this position you can perform massage for yourself without fighting the pull of gravity on body fluids, although you may find this rather tiring.

Adolescent arch strain. After either an athletic event or a day which involves unusual amounts of standing and walking, teenagers and young adults sometimes get pain along the inner and lower margins of the arch. There may be slight swelling and tenderness in this area, but there should not be tenderness at any spot along the bones of the top of the foot. Bony tenderness sometimes points toward so-called "march fractures"—tiny cracks in the bones which occur with prolonged hiking, especially over rough ground—and these require a doctor's care. Otherwise arch pain usually responds to home measures.

Contrast baths, as described on page 29, give some immediate relief. In some instances, a well-fitting hunter's boot or other firm, solid-soled shoe will give enough support. It is best to wear such shoes all the time rather than go barefoot or switch to soft slippers, since the shoe's sole acts as a splint. If these measures do not control discomfort, the foot will have to be strapped with adhesive tape.

Tricks for taping. Try to avoid waterproof tape if possible—it traps sweat underneath and peels off more quickly. Shave off any long hairs, which will otherwise cause discomfort when the tape is removed. The tape will stick better and cause less irritation if you paint the skin underneath with tincture of benzoin (available at any drugstore without prescription). Let this coat dry thoroughly before beginning the tape job.

There are several tricks you can use to apply adhesive tape smoothly to any body part. Measure the approximate length of a strip by unrolling it and laying the back of the tape (not the sticky side) against the skin. At the same time, you can check the way the tape will follow body contours, making it easier to wind up the right place when you apply it "for keeps." Cut several strips at a time and apply them from the middle rather than from one end, smoothing the tape into place without pulling or stretching it, with the direction determined entirely by body contours. Overlap strips by 1/3 their width—narrow gaps between strips, which sometimes occur when you cut your margins too close, cut painfully with the least swelling. If it is practical, apply an elastic bandage over your tape job for a few hours at least—tape sticks much better if it is kept in close contact with the skin until it is thoroughly warm.

Tape for arch strain. Use 1-inch tape cut to lengths of 15 to 18 inches. Have the patient turn his or her foot outward (toward the little toe side) as far as possible. Angle the middle of one piece of tape across the inner side of the heel and smooth it into contact with the skin in both directions. One end should wind up on the top of the arch, coming up from its outer rim. The other should come around the outside of the ankle and end at or near the junction of the top of the foot and the ankle. Place three or four additional strips parallel to the first, overlapping about 1/3 of the tape width.

Now have the patient turn the foot inward as far as possible. The tape already applied should hold the heel in an outward-rolled position, so that this movement should have the effect of increasing the height of the arch and relieving strain on its ligaments. Start the middle of a piece of tape along the bottom of the foot near the bases of the toes. The ends should follow the foot contours in a spiral up the arch, joining (at some rather unpredictable point) the tape already applied to the heel. Apply three or four further overlapping strips behind the first. It is more important to keep the tape smooth and apply it without pull than it is to get it to go in the right direction. To finish covering the entire foot, use either a spiral of tape or a series of encircling strips around the arch, applied smoothly and without tension.

This tape should be left in place for a week or ten days, or reapplied in the same fashion if it becomes either loose or intolerably dirty.

Long-range help with arch troubles. If you have painful or weak arches, here's a step-by-step approach to your long-range problem:

1. Get oxford-type shoes that fit your arch properly by following the four steps outlined above.

2. If you still have discomfort, get cork shoe inserts to prop up the crucial parts of your arch. Do these two foot exercises daily for three weeks:

> Pick up one dozen ¾ inch marbles with the toes of each foot, and deposit them in a hat or box.
> Stand on your toes in your bare feet. Turn your ankles about halfway inward. Roll your weight slowly down along the outside of your feet until it rests on your heels. Repeat ten times.

3. If this gives relief most of the time, control occasional discomfort after special strain with contrast baths (detailed directions on page 29).

4. If you continue to have trouble and are over age forty, get rigid plastic or steel and leather arch supports. Such supports give comfort at the price of weakening your foot muscles and making your need for arch supports likely to increase. But they *do* give comfort, which makes them worthwhile when other measures have failed.

Joggers' foot. Probably the most common misery that drives people off the jogging track is pain across the foot at the base of the toes. This condition usually comes from strain of the cross-wise arch. In addition to your main arch under the middle of the foot, you have a series of ligaments which hold the front of the foot bones in stable position with the center bones slightly farther off the ground than the end ones. Jogging puts extra strain on these structures, and often stretches the ligaments so that they no longer do the job. You can test yourself for this condition very easily by placing your index fingers under the edges of the front of your foot and pressing down on the center of the top of your foot with both thumbs. If you can push the center of the front end of your foot down until it bulges toward the sole, your crosswise arch has failed.

When this condition causes substantial pain or discomfort, use contrast baths as described above. As soon as the pain has settled down, get a metatarsal pad which fits under the front ends of the second and third foot bones. Dr. Scholl's makes a very simple device that is held in place by a loop around your big toe. The leather insoles described above also work very well, at somewhat higher cost. Be sure to get some good, well fitted jogger's shoes which are loose enough to let you wear two pairs of athletic socks. No guarantees—once the arch has collapsed there's a good chance that your running days are over. But these measures work as well as anything I know (except perhaps switching to swimming).

Bunions. When the ball of your foot splays out at the base of your big toe, pressure against the side of your shoe often causes swelling and pain. You can usually get relief from such discomfort with contrast baths and aspirin. To keep the bunions from getting worse and ultimately requiring operation, these further steps are worthwhile:

1. Get at least one pair of low heeled lacing oxfords for everyday wear, and have your shoemaker attach an anterior heel, which is a block of leather toward the front of the arch which spreads your weight to the foot bones instead of letting it roll up on the ball of your foot with each stride.

2. Stick to low or medium heels even for dress-up occasions. High heels more than double the weight on the front of the foot, which definitely makes bunions worse.

Ingrown toenail. Home care usually relieves ingrown toenail temporarily, and sometimes gives a permanent cure. If a deep spur, severe infection, or some health problem like diabetes complicates the problem, best see your doctor right away. Otherwise try these home measures:

1. Hot soaks. The corner of your nail usually digs in enough to cause redness, swelling and pain before you realize that anything is wrong. Hot soaks for 20 minutes three or four times a day help to take the redness and swelling out.

2. Side and center trimming. As soon as hot soaks have settled down the tenderness to allow relatively pain-free handling, you want to remove the corner of the toenail which is digging into your flesh. While the nail is still soft after a soak, clean the toe with alcohol. Wash your hands thoroughly. Rest the toe against a firm surface like the top of a footstool or low table. Peel the fold of skin off the base of the nail with an orange stick or the end of a fingernail file. With a clean, new, single edged razor blade, make a cut part way through the nail, begining at the side of the nail just above its base and cutting straight toward the tip of the toe. Start far enough down to leave a long, smooth incline which will push the skin back as the nail grows out. Deepen this cut until the fragment of nail which has dug in is nearly free. With manicure scissors and tweezers, free up the loose portion and remove it. In the same way, remove a narrow pie-shaped wedge from the center of the nail with its base at the nail end and its point about halfway up the nail. This makes the edge of the nail more yielding and improves your chance of getting the nail corner to grow out past the skin instead of digging in. As the nail grows out, soak the toe and recut this pie-shaped wedge at intervals.

3. Petroleum jelly corner-lifting packs. You can keep the advancing corner of the nail from digging in by pushing a small piece of petroleum jelly impregnated gauze underneath it daily. Unravel a roll of one inch roller gauze into a wide mouthed jar. Add about one ounce of petroleum jelly. Heat uncovered in a warm oven for thirty minutes. The melted petroleum jelly will impregnate the gauze. For use, cut off a small piece of the gauze and pack it under the advancing corner of the toenail with a toothpick or small finishing nail. The petroleum jelly keeps the nail more yielding, and the packing helps lift it out of the flesh.

4. Get shoes with extra toe room. If you have ever had ingrown nails, you need shoes with a straight inner margin instead of pointed toes, and preferably with a box or a moccasin type front.

Thickened and deformed nails. If you have very heavy toenails or very sharply arched nails which dig into your toe from shoe pressure on the top, frequent trimming and filing may help. Always soak the nails for 20 minutes before attempting to cut them, or wait until you have taken a long, soaking tub bath. Clippers work much better than scissors on this type of nail. The straight-cut variety of clippers can be obtained in most drugstores for about two dollars. An ordinary file or piece of coarse sandpaper often works better than any other measure to thin the nail or relieve pressure. File away at the top of the nail, not at the end. Be sure that you do not cut the corners too far back, because this kind of nail very easily becomes ingrown.

2

Surprising Results Using Home Measures for Low Blood Sugar and Food Allergy

When I first started in country practice, I almost killed off a couple of my patients. Back in the city, I had always told patients who needed medicine three times a day to take it "before each meal." But farm folk use the big muscles of their backs and legs hour after hour and burn up a lot of fuel. So they eat more often. Besides breakfast, dinner and supper, many farm families have mid-morning and mid-afternoon "lunch"—so "before each meal" turned out to be *five* doses instead of *three*.

If you don't let a city-bred doctor kill you off with an overdose of pills, there's some reason to think that this eating pattern does a lot of good. Both the steady sturdiness and the phlegmatic, contented mood which typify farm folk may well stem as much from their eating pattern as from their active and independent way of life. Or, to look at the other side of the coin, much of the weariness, irritability, physical miseries and depression which less active people suffer may result from less frequent meals and resulting blood sugar ups and downs.

DOES HYPOGLYCEMIA CAUSE ANY PROBLEMS FOR YOU?

Doctors have known for years that certain complaints come from low blood sugar. Patients who suffered from headaches, dizzy spells, fainting or weakness late in the morning or afternoon generally have had blood chemistry tests which showed low sugar as the cause. But this part of the hypoglycemia problem is only the tip of the iceberg: many more people, perhaps one out of four, suffer from loss of concentration, depression, craving for alcohol or sweets, irritability and other vague complaints because of low blood sugar.

Years before medical science had any inkling of it, some "ordinary folks" really pinpointed this condition. Ask any schoolmarm which period she least likes to teach and she'll specify the last in the morning or the last in the afternoon when the kids are fractious and irritable, can't concentrate and won't behave. Computer-aided studies in college show the same thing—all students average poorer grades in the last period before lunch, and those who don't eat breakfast dip a full letter grade below their own average in this period.

Irritability and inability to concentrate when your blood sugar is low stem from one fact: your brain and nervous system have no reserves of fuel and function only when they have the right amount of sugar available to burn. Muscles have stores of glycogen which your body can change to sugar in case of need, inner organs can burn fat or convert protein to sugars at will. But your brain and nervous system depend completely on the steady supply of glucose in your body fluids and work at par only when the glucose level is above 65 mgms %.

So why do some people have hypoglycemia while others don't?

The usual kink in the works has to do with sugar storage. When you eat, your body soaks in sugar faster than it burns it up. Your blood sugar rises to a certain level, then your body starts up mechanisms that turn the extra sugar into glycogen and store it, mainly in your liver. When your blood sugar drops below a certain point, your body flips this mechanism into reverse. The lucky people who never suffer from hypoglycemia change from storing glycogen to *calling up reserves* as soon as the after-meal surplus is taken care of. But if you have hypoglycemia, your body doesn't react that quickly to blood sugar drop. It keeps storing sugar for extra hours, pulling your blood level down into the miserable fifties or the dangerous forties, leaving key brain cells starved for fuel and unable to function.

Thus the paradox: the worst thing for a person with low blood sugar is a high sugar meal. Waffles and syrup or sweet rolls or ice cream sundaes make him feel just great at the time, but the rebound two or three hours later puts him in the dumps. And that's the first clue you should look for in deciding whether *you* have a hypoglycemia problem: big swings in energy level, mood or intellectual capability. Especially if you hit bottom in any of those ways in late morning and late afternoon.

A self-testing technique for hypoglycemia. If you have those wide swings in energy level or in mood or in thinking capacity, or if you have specific complaints such as headache, dizziness, cold sweats and washed-out fatigue, you can often tell whether or not they are hypoglycemic by a simple self-test. Do the complaints disappear almost instantly when you drink a glass of orange juice or eat a few soft mints? This test is particularly helpful with distinct complaints such as headache or washed-out fatigue. Sonya J., for instance, had suffered from these complaints for many years without identifying the source. When she tried the "soft mints cure," on one of her headaches, she got complete relief in ninety seconds. She started to carry quickly-absorbed sweets with her everywhere, and tried them on several complaints. When she suddenly "gave out" during a tennis game, she decided to try "quick energy" sweets and regained her zoom in two minutes.

As we'll see shortly, sweets are *not* the basis of long-range control because of later rebound. But any symptom that disappears entirely in five minutes or less when you take something sweet is almost certainly hypo-glycemic in origin. You don't need blood chemistry tests to know you're hypoglycemic if sugar gives a dramatic cure.

Subtle forms of hypoglycemia. Unfortunately, this test isn't always clear-cut when vaguer symptoms like altered mood, sugar and alcohol craving and loss of concentration are involved. If wide swings in these qualities make you suspect hypoglycemia, you have two choices:

1. Try the hypoglycemia diet outlined below for a week, and see how much better you feel. If the diet works, what more do you need to know?

2. If you want to get on "solid scientific ground," fast from midnight until breakfast time, drink super-sweet lemonade with five or more table-spoonsful of sugar in it for breakfast, and have your doctor check your blood sugar exactly four hours later. No other food or fluids (except water) in the meanwhile, of course. If your sugar is below 65, especially if it is substantially below that level, get on that hypoglycemia diet and stay there! I'll bet dollars to doughnuts (or is that good odds these days?) that you'll feel substantially better if you do, whether or not your own doctor calls the test "normal."

The hypoglycemia diet. Meat, fish, eggs and cheese, all of which contain lots of protein, are the mainstays of a sugar-curve-smoothing diet. Proteins help in two ways: first, they don't kick off the pendulum—while sugars and starches send blood glucose high enough to start a rebound, proteins soak in slowly. Second, a large portion of the protein you eat converts very slowly to carbohydrate. This slow drip of available blood sugar fills in the trough in your curve and keeps you from ever being fully depleted. There's also an incidental benefit from working lots of protein into a hypoglycemia diet—if you're eating several extra times a day, weight gain can become a problem, and protein foods have less impact on your weight than fats or carbohydrates.

So you want to work lots of protein into your hypoglycemia-fighting program. The first and major principle is *protein foods at each meal*, at least three times a day. Most people automatically include protein in their evening meal, so breakfast and lunch are the meals you have to concentrate on. If you like eggs, they're super for breakfast—inexpensive, quickly prepared and very rich in protein. Ham and Canadian bacon also fill the bill. Sausage and bacon aren't quite as good, because they have more fat and calories per unit of protein, but they satisfy the need if you render out most of the fat in cooking. So-called "high protein cereals" are a snare and a delusion—none of them even comes close to the recommended foods in ratio of protein to calories. For lunch try cottage cheese, tuna fish salad, chicken or turkey salad, Edam, Gouda or Provolone cheese as "main dishes." Or if you prefer the sandwich route, eat one very thickly filled one rather than two or more thinly-filled ones (since the filling is usually high in protein and the extra bread is not).

Although three high protein meals a day usually smooth out the blood sugar level fairly well, many people need small between-meals snacks to reach their ideal functioning level. I usually ask my patients to follow a rigid six-feeding pattern for two weeks or so to see how good they can feel, then drop as many of the between-meals snacks as they find dispensable. Protein foods make the best between-meal snacks, too. Since you won't always be at home when the need arises, it's best to use foods which don't require refrigeration. Chipped beef, corned beef, pastrami and beef jerky, ham, smoked pork, Thuringer, cervelat and summer sausage are the main available meats. If you use Thuringer, cervelat or summer sausage, slice it fairly thin and broil slightly on both sides. Most of the fat will render out and can be blotted off with a paper towel. Tastes great warm, but still tastes good after riding around in your purse or pocket (inside a plastic bag) most of the day.

Ciscoes, smoked fish (in several varieties), and marinated herring also meet this need. Sardines in mustard or tomato sauce will stay fresh for a few hours in a plastic container, and have all the protein without the extra fat of the oil-packed varieties. Water-pack tuna is cheap and good, but requires refrigeration. The same is true of cottage cheese, while the cheeses made from whole or partly skimmed milk (like Edam, Gouda, and pro-volone) last for days and taste better at room temperature than cold. Where possible weight gain is a problem, I would avoid the high fat cheeses like Swiss and cheddar. Boiled eggs last without refrigeration, but if you get fancy and devil them or make egg salad you should use a cooler.

With a normal morning-noon-night meal schedule, snacks at 10:30, 3:30 and 9 are ideal. You can adapt this program to your own schedule very easily if you simply space the six feedings out fairly evenly through your waking hours. After the first two weeks, try dropping one snack after another until you find the minimum program which keeps you feeling tops. Most patients get down to three or four feedings, but a few need to stay close to the full program for life.

A few "don'ts" go along with these "do's." Concentrated sweets or starches kick off the hypoglycemia pendulum and then give big trouble two or three hours later, so candy, desserts, or straight starches often cause later distress. That doesn't mean that you can never have a dessert—just eat it along with a substantial protein meal, never as a between-meal snack. Hot cakes, waffles and syrup, spaghetti or other pasta (unless heavily mixed with meat-containing sauce), macaroni and other heavy-starch-with-no-protein meals often cause later rebound and should be avoided. Caffeine in coffee seems to cause more trouble to people with hypoglycemia than to others. I usually tell patients to drink Sanka or Brim when they brew their own, so that what they get at restaurants or away from home won't be piled on an already-high caffeine base.

Anything which enters so deeply into everyday decisions, such as when to eat what, seems to be a lot of bother. Nevertheless, I have literally hundreds of patients who feel enough better on a hypoglycemia program to stick with it year after year. Take Nancy M., for instance.

"Sure, I've fallen off the wagon once in a while," she said. "What can you do when you're at a party and the hostess serves a gorgeous dessert? But then it hits me afterwards, and I go right back on the program."

"So you've been sticking to the diet for three years?"

"That's right. And I haven't had a headache or dizzy spell as long as I follow the rules. But the main thing I've noticed is my mood—I don't yell at the kids any more, or get the blues, or feel spaced out. Just living on an even keel—that's what makes it worthwhile for me."

Severe forms of hypoglycemia. Low blood sugar after a fast is different from rebound hypoglycemia and sometimes is the result of an insulin-producing tumor. While such tumors are very rare, anyone who has hypoglycemic symptoms before breakfast or who gets worse after fasting should have further tests. Hypoglycemia also occurs with certain diseases of the liver, so accompanying indigestion, gas, jaundice or abdominal swelling show need for a medical examination. Hypoglycemia also occurs in some patients who are taking insulin or other drugs for diabetes, and calls for changes in management of that disease.

A few of my patients with classic (but unusually severe) hypoglycemia have been found to have lower-than-normal adrenal hormone levels and have benefited from hormone injections. You should see a doctor for special tests if your symptoms seem characteristic but fail to respond to diet alone.

With these few exceptions, self-diagnosis and self-treatment of hypoglycemia is safe and effective. If you have any reason to suspect this condition in yourself, follow the program outlined above. It's quite likely to give truly surprising results—to uncover a more energetic, stable and happier "you" that never before existed!

FOOD ALLERGY

Table talk in my physician-father's house was sometimes hard on the squeamish person, but often proved educational. For instance, a guest in our house when I was a youngster suddenly excused himself from the dinner table after learning that the soup he was eating contained shrimp. He returned slightly pale but cheerful. Because everyone present (except me at the time) was involved in medicine, he felt free to discuss his problem.

"Even one bite of shrimp gives me cramps and diarrhea for a day or more," he said. "So if I eat some without realizing it, I just tickle the back of my throat until I throw up. It's a bit unpleasant, but it's over within five minutes that way."

That's the kind of food allergy which has been recognized for many years—distinct and sudden symptoms, usually cramps and watery diarrhea without the accompanying fever, dragged out feeling, headache or aches and pains which comes with food infection. It is generally traced to an uncommonly eaten food such as shellfish, citron, nuts or a special seasoning. But like the classic low blood sugar syndrome, this pattern has proved to be the merest tip of the iceberg, with subtler forms of food allergy among the commonest ailments of mankind. Food allergy causes or aggravates all of the following complaints:

Headache.
Upset stomach, loss of appetite, diarrhea, cramps, vomiting.
Chronic or recurrent hives or eczema, superficial skin swellings.
Rapid pulse, light-headedness, dizziness.
Pink eye or conjunctivitis.
Postnasal drip, nasal congestion, sinus blockage.
Fatigue and weakness.
Asthma and hay fever.

Urinary frequency.
Irritability and mood swings, hyperactivity.
Childhood feeding problems.
Sleep disturbances.

Moreover, the foods which most commonly cause allergy are not the rare treats like shrimp and citron. Those were merely recognized because the victim ate them so seldom that he could quickly associate them with his later symptoms. The worst offenders are the everday foods—wheat, milk, eggs, and the bean family (including coffee, chocolate from cocoa beans, soy sauce which is made from the soya bean, and peanuts, which belong to the bean family rather than the nut family). Almost every wholesome food you can name, including meat, fish, most vegetables and almost all fruits have been proved to cause allergic symptoms in some people. About the only foods known which rarely or never cause allergy are rice, lamb and salt.

How to tell if you have a food allergy. The patients for whom I have detected food allergies fall into two groups: First, those whose symptoms distinctly suggest allergy, the sufferers from headaches, hives, asthma, nasal congestion or postnasal drip, recurrent diarrhea or vomiting, and rapid pulse. Paradoxically, the worse the symptoms are the easier it is to find the allergies—complaints clear up altogether when the offending foods are eliminated and return with a vengeance when the offending foods are deliberately restored. If you have any of these symptoms, try one of the two "major detection methods" described below.

Second, many people have vaguer complaints or no complaints at all—the latter because they have had their symptoms so long that they don't have any standard for comparison. They feel as well as they have always felt, so they don't express any complaints, but after they find and eliminate their allergies, they come back and say: "I just didn't know how good I could feel." This has happened often enough in my experience that I recommend the "major detection methods" to anyone who doesn't feel absolutely confident in his or her blooming state of health. If those methods seem too extreme, you should at least try the "minor methods" for a week or so just on the chance that you'll find something of great benefit to you without ever knowing that you have a problem.

The major detection methods. First and foremost, don't depend on allergy tests of any kind for the detection of food allergy. If you actually suffer from this disorder, the chances are that your body is reacting to one of the breakdown products of the offending food rather than to the protein in its original, intact form. Thus you can show no reaction whatever to a skin test with wheat extract and still have symptoms every time you eat anything made with wheat flour. A great many doctors, particularly specialists in allergy, still use these expensive and uncomfortable tests, but in my opinion they are utterly worthless. A self-administered home program works very much better at absolutely no cost.

The fast. While I very seldom recommend a total fast for the purpose of detecting food allergies, I've still made the diagnosis quite often by inquiring as to the effects of a fast. Even eating habits can give a tip off—if a patient tells me that he skips breakfast and often skips lunch, careful inquiry often shows that he's fallen into this pattern because he "feels better"—has more energy, can concentrate better, gets more accomplished. In some instances, patients have initially fasted for religious reasons or because of necessity, and found that they feel so much better after a day or two that they continue to fast periodically "to clear out the poisons." In some instances, radical weight loss programs become almost equivalent to a fast—when the "Last Chance Diet" with predigested protein was in style many people who found that they felt better on this program proved to have food allergies. And patients who voluntarily fast for weight control often submit themselves to this ordeal because relief of allergic symptoms balances off against the miseries of hunger and makes the experience much more bearable.

In ideal circumstances—when you can stand to lose a few pounds, when you won't be called upon to operate machinery or do anything else which would make dizziness (a frequent complication of fasting) risky, and when food deprival hasn't proved too hard for you to take—a three day fast should relieve virtually all food-allergy-related symptoms you might have. Plain water won't hurt these results, but any other food or fluid, even those you've always taken without "having them cause you any trouble," should be eliminated. This test works very well with one exception: if the allergy-caused symptoms resemble those which stem from fasting itself, such as dizziness and weakness, the lamb and rice test is much to be preferred.

The lamb and rice test. Rather than suffer the rigors of a total fast, most patients prefer the culinary horrors of a rice and lamb diet. Since practically nobody is allergic to these two foods, or to ordinary table salt and drinking water, allergic symptoms virtually always disappear when you eat these foods *and nothing else.* Generally it takes about three days to complete a valid test, since the process of digestion takes as much as 48 hours. A four or five day test works better if you also suffer from constipation, so that remnants of the offending food remain in your system a bit longer. When complaints are sporadic—bursting headaches every few days, for instance—you may need to stay on the rice and lamb bit for several extra days to be sure that the problem has really disappeared.

How Lydia Pierce cured her food allergies. Lydia Pierce's main complaints were fatigue and inability to concentrate, but as soon as I took a detailed history another interesting fact emerged: For the past two years, she had passed eight to ten watery stools each day. This amount of diarrhea almost always causes fatigue, because it washes so much sodium and potassium out of your system that you suffer from depletion of these much-needed electrolytes. That's why you get your energy back more quickly after a bout of diarrhea if you eat heavily-salted soups and potassium-rich fruit juices than if you go back on a normal diet.

"I've noticed that," Lydia said, when I explained the connection between her fatigue and her diarrhea. "I do feel better when I get a lot of salt. But I thought too much salt would be bad for me."

"If you're taking it to make up for excess loss, it can't do you any harm. But why don't we try for something a little more permanent, like getting rid of the diarrhea altogether?"

"That would be great. But I've tried everything from Kaopectate to spasm soothers, and nothing does the trick."

At this point, I explained the rice and lamb diet to Lydia, and she agreed to try it. In one day her diarrhea cleared up completely, and she felt like a new woman.

What to do if fasting on the rice and lamb diet helps you. The next step in your home food allergy cure is to identify exactly which foods cause your trouble. To do this, you simply add two new foods—one from the high-risk and one from the low-risk list—each three days. When symptoms recur, you've probably found an offender. Lydia's case worked out that way— she felt perfectly well until she added eggs, then the diarrhea instantly recurred. Now she carefully avoids eggs in any form, including foods (like cake and pasta) in which eggs are used as an ingredient, and she has very little diarrhea or fatigue. In order to get back to a fairly balanced diet quickly, I advise adding foods in this order, with the high risk food in each pair identified by an asterisk:

1. Milk* (and all dairy products) plus grapefruit.
2. Wheat* (including bread, anything containing flour, and certain breakfast cereals) plus beef.
3. Eggs* (and anything using eggs as an ingredient) plus cauliflower.
4. Beans* (including coffee, chocolate, soy sauce and peanuts) plus pork (including ham and bacon).
5. Tomato* plus lettuce.
6. Your favorite shellfish* (shrimp, scallops, oysters or clams) plus pears.

From here on, add foods two at a time in any order. Remember that different species—whitefish, bass and trout for instance—are each separate allergens, so that you can't assume that if one variety of fish, vegetable or fruit doesn't cause trouble another variety will also prove innocent. And if you have one major allergy, such as wheat or eggs, chances are that you will also prove to have allergies to several other types of food. When you have "struck oil" by discovering one thing that consistently causes your symptoms, you still need to carry through the rest of the program. Eliminate the wheat (or whatever), then go on adding two foods at a time until you have covered almost everything in the index of your cookbook. Lydia Pierce, for instance, got rid of most of her complaints when she eliminated eggs, but she still had occasional headaches and stomach upsets which we finally traced to secondary allergies—in her case tomatoes, strawberries and citron.

The reason "secondary allergies" almost always develop is simple. During an allergic attack your stomach and intestinal lining become inflamed and engorged, allowing chemicals which ordinarily could not get into your bloodstream in an undigested form to penetrate. Thus the "main allergy" opens the door for proteins and polypeptides to reach your liver through the bloodstream. Your liver makes antibodies to almost any foreign substance that comes to it through the blood, and whenever those antibodies meet the substance to which they originally formed you get an allergic reaction. I have found secondary allergies in almost every patient who definitely had food allergy, and therefore recommend a diligent further search even after the main allergen has been identified. Keep adding to your original rice-lamb-water-salt program until you have really checked out all the foods you commonly encounter, and then try the pulse test approach after every meal for several months to see if you can catch any minor offenders you might still have missed. It's a lot of work and a lot of bother, but if you nail down every single allergen, you'll feel better than you have in years, often ridding yourself of a dozen minor complaints which you never suspected of being allergic.

Minor detection methods. A few of my patients have been able to identify important food allergies with two methods that are much simpler than the elimination diet or fast. These methods are not as reliable and I usually recommend them only for the late stage of "allergen chasing," when you have spotted the main problem foods and are dotting the i's and crossing the t's. But if your allergies are relatively minor, or if only minor "secondary allergies" remain after you have followed the program recommended above, the pulse test and the food diary approach deserve a try.

The pulse test. An allergic reaction almost always causes an increase in your pulse rate, along with the other disruptions in the way your system functions. If the offending food soaks into your system quickly and if the allergic reaction occurs to the food protein itself (or a very early breakdown product), the resulting pulse rise gives a reliable clue.

That's how Glen Maxwell discovered his coffee allergy, for instance. Glen had no idea that anything was wrong with him—actually he came to my office for an insurance examination. But his heart was banging away at a rate over 100 (against an average of 72 for men or 80 for women).

"Any chance it's just from too much coffee?" I asked him.

"Could be. I usually demolish a pot or so when I'm sitting around the office in the morning."

"Well, that's one thing you can certainly check for yourself, and possibly avoid a lot of expensive medical tests in the process. Just count your pulse first thing in the morning, then check again about a half hour after breakfast. If your pulse speeds up more than 8 beats a minute, chances are you have some form of extra sensitivity—either over-response to caffeine or allergy to the coffee bean."

"But how do I count my own pulse?"

"Just turn your head to the right and lay your first two fingers on your neck just below the angle of your jaw on the left. You'll feel the carotid artery thumping away under the edge of the neck muscles. Count the beats for 15 seconds and multiply by four."

Glen called the next morning to say that his breakfast coffee kicked up his pulse rate by 12 beats.

"In that case," I told him, "either you're unduly sensitive to caffeine (so that you should avoid coffee, tea and cola drinks) or you're allergic to the bean family (in which case you should avoid coffee, chocolate, peanuts and all forms of beans)."

"How do I tell which?" he asked.

"Try the same test tomorrow with Brim or Sanka. If your pulse speeds up from decaffeinated brands, you can be pretty sure that it's a true food allergy rather than an overreaction to stimulants."

And that's what it proved to be. A few weeks later, Glen called to thank me for pointing it out to him.

"I feel like a new man," he said. "Lots more energy, feel sharper, less irritable—I didn't know what that stuff was doing to me all these years."

You can use this same test to check for some food allergies. Just check your pulse first thing in the morning and again half an hour after each meal or snack (including beverages). This test only shows up the immediate reactions, and as mentioned above many allergic reactions come on slowly. But it's very helpful in detecting coffee sensitivity, and it often helps to identify the secondary allergens that you encounter too rarely to catch with your elimination diet program.

The food diary. "Every spring I get this crazy rash," Harry Johnson said. "And the funny thing is it always happens during Lent and disappears at Easter."

"That's a new one," I remarked, "a religious rash. Well, let's take a look."

He had red, raised, itchy spots, mainly on the trunk and upper extremities. It looked like an allergic reaction to me, but careful questioning disclosed no medication, chemical exposure, or other probable source.

"Probably a food allergy," I told him as I wrote out a prescription for an ointment to give temporary relief. "Why don't you write down everything you eat or drink for a couple of days, and we'll see if we can get some idea of what might be causing it. I'm particularly interested in what you eat within a day or so before any new flare-up of the rash, so make a note too of times when the itching seems worse."

Actually, we didn't have to go the full route with Harry. As soon as he began writing down everything he ate, one item stood out like a neon sign: during Lent the place where he ate lunch every day served hot cross buns, and Harry easily proved to himself that the citron in them caused his allergy. The rash disappeared when he omitted the buns, and recurred when he ate a small amount of citron as a deliberate test.

If you have a distinct allergic symptom of any kind, keeping a food diary might help you to "put two and two together" the way Harry did. Just remember that the flare in symptoms can occur any time in the 48 hours after consuming the offending food or beverage. It can be immediate, but symptoms can also occur quite abruptly after a substantial delay (when the process of food breakdown finally reaches the stage which makes the substance you are sensitive to).

Doctors and food allergy. As mentioned above, the traditional method of skin testing for allergy does not work well for food allergies. A relatively new and complicated test called the "Ig E" (for a specific fraction of immune globulin) generally is positive when any food allergy is present. This test is quite expensive (about $35) and is not 100% accurate, but I have found it helpful in some cases when results of the home methods discussed above were not conclusive.

If you discover that you have numerous food allergies, you may find that the foods you can eat without causing symptoms no longer allow a very well rounded diet. A patient who is allergic to milk, for instance, almost always winds up eating much less calcium than his body needs. This particular deficiency becomes especially troublesome in the event of pregnancy or in women who have passed the menopause (and are therefore subject to bone-weakening osteoporosis, discussed in another chapter). If there is any question in your mind that your self-designed allergy diet might be deficient in some mineral or vitamin, check with your physician or with a qualified nutritionist.

Finally, always remember that you can get "fleas and lice both"—that a proven allergic origin of certain symptoms doesn't mean that nothing else is wrong. If any of your symptoms suggest serious disease, don't delay the checkups you need until you can get around to proving whether or not they are allergic. And if some symptoms remain after you have controlled part of your problem with an allergy diet, don't just assume that you have further allergies but haven't yet identified them. Patients with food allergies can get all the other things the human tribe is subject to, from ulcers and tumors to appendicitis and hemmorrhage. Take care of the "fleas" yourself, but don't fail to call your doctor if there's any reason to suspect "lice."

THE GIST OF THIS CHAPTER

Low blood sugar can cause a host of complaints, ranging from headaches and dizziness to mood swings and inability to concentrate. Any such difficulties which tend to recur in the late morning and late afternoon should make you suspect low blood sugar. If you get prompt relief from such a complaint when you eat a soft mint or drink a glass of orange juice, you'll probably find it worthwhile to follow a full hypoglycemia program for two weeks.

The mainstay of a hypoglycemia-curing diet is protein. Include meat, fish, cheese and eggs in every meal, and spread your food intake through six spaced feedings a day. Although "sweets" might seem the common-sense remedy for low blood sugar, later rebound makes them do much more harm than good. Except when used for a short emergency "lift" or as tests to see if certain complaints are hypoglycemic, you should avoid concentrated sugars and starches.

Food allergies can also cause a wide variety of complaints, ranging from vomiting and cramps to headaches, skin rashes, stuffy nose, asthma and fatigue. Three self-testing procedures—a brief fast, the rice and lamb diet and the pulse test—will help you to discover and identify your food allergies. Even if you've never recognized that you have a problem (which most sufferers don't, because they don't have a standard for comparison), finding and eliminating your food allergies may make you feel like a new person.

3

Home Remedies for
Arthritis and Rheumatism

If Minnesotans weren't so blasted stoical, they would eat aspirin by the ton for creaking joints. The hard physical work of farming and forestry plus plenty of he-man outdoor recreation puts lots of strain on North Country spines and joints. We have more than our share of arthritics here. My patients have had more than enough chance to try various home remedies and correctives for arthritis, aching joints, bursitis, and other forms of rheumatism. Here are the measures they've found most effective through the years:

HOME MEASURES FOR JOINT PAINS

Whether you suffer from stiff fingers, painful joints or full-blown arthritic disease, joint trouble gives you real misery. Don't rely entirely on home measures for any substantial degree of arthritis—prescription medicines these days give so much relief and protection from crippling that you would be foolish to pass them up. Most of the patients who used to have to choose between living with their miseries and risking major-league complications from powerful drugs like the cortisones now get substantial relief from Motrin or Tolectin, which have very few side effects. Indocin gives tremendous benefit in some cases, although you do need to check with your doctor frequently while you take it because of occasional dangerous effect on your blood cells. I have even seen patients apparently cured of severe rheumatoid arthritis with Cupramine; one person was free of symptoms and off all medication after five years. Even a few years ago, when the last edition of this book came out, such results would have looked like miracles, but today they are more the rule than the exception.

Still, home measures often help, both for minor joint pains which simply don't justify expensive doctor care and to supplement the new prescription measures. You can often get complete relief with simple home care, and these measures are perfectly safe, as long as you don't stick with them when continued difficulty really calls for an all-out attack.

Red, swollen joints. Active joint disease with swelling, redness, heat and pain calls for gentle, soothing measures. Intense heat, massage, or exercise merely adds to the congestion and makes the situation worse. At this stage, these techniques usually provide most helpful:

The hormone-stimulating aspirin dose. Doctors have known for years that aspirin relieves joint and muscle aches much more completely if you take it according to a certain dosage pattern: high doses the first day or two, with smaller but still regular doses thereafter. Recently they found out why this is true. Used in high starting, steady doses, aspirin definitely spurs your body to form safe amounts of cortisone and its hormone cousins—the great new miracle drugs that have put even crippled, bedridden victims of arthritis back on their feet! You can get the benefit of medicine's strongest treatment for your joint and muscle aches simply by taking aspirin according to this plan:

> Take aspirin tablets on arising, after breakfast, lunch, and supper, and at bedtime. The number of tablets at each dose depends upon your weight. If you weigh 100–135 pounds, take 2 tablets at each dose for a total of ten tablets daily. If you weigh 136–170 pounds, take 3 tablets at each dose for a total of fifteen tablets daily. If you weigh over 170 pounds, take three tablets on arising and at bedtime and four tablets after each meal for a total of eighteen tablets daily.
>
> Continue this dosage for three days or until you feel considerably better. Then drop the morning dose, continuing the other four doses daily. Continue to take the tablets regularly, even if you need them over a period of years. If you think you need less medicine, take one less tablet for your evening dose, wait three days and if still feeling well cut another of your doses, and so on.

A lot of people worry about whether aspirin will subtly undermine their blood or general health when used over a period of months or years. The answer is, *absolutely no,* if you never take it on an empty stomach. Any harmful effects which have been reported stem from blood seepage within the stomach, caused by the irritating effect of undiluted aspirin lying directly against the stomach wall. Unless aspirin causes clear-cut distress, the program recommended above is entirely harmless. If you get heartburn or nausea after taking aspirin, take it after meals, drink milk instead of water with each pill, or switch to either buffered aspirin or coated tablets of sodium salicylate (which don't dissolve until they get through your stomach). If you still get nauseated, or if you get dizzy from aspirin, you're the one person in several thousand who is allergic to it and has to use other means of relief.

Red joints in children. Red, swollen joints often signal rheumatic fever rather than simple joint disease in children, adolescents and young adults. The larger joints—knees, ankles and elbows—are more likely to be involved than smaller ones. One joint will usually flare, then clear up in a day or two, with other joints flaring up in succession. Victims often have some fever, but may have a normal temperature. Since rheumatic fever can present quite varied symptoms in different cases and may involve the heart, it is always wise to get a doctor in on the case right away whenever you even suspect that this condition *might* be present.

Warm flannel. You can usually get some relief from swollen-joint pain with warm flannel wrappings. The easiest method is to wrap or cover the joint with two or three layers of flannel and cover loosely with a heating pad set for low heat. Remove or shift the pad as the flannel reaches a cozy warmth. Keep the joint lightly warmed for about an hour at a time, three or more times a day.

Diet. Two of the three common forms of joint trouble respond to shifts in diet. Rheumatoid arthritis, which usually starts in people who have not yet turned 40 and tends to leave stiffened joints in the wake of each attack, seems to improve somewhat on a *low residue diet*. Omit raw vegetables, cabbage, brussels sprouts, broccoli, and bran cereals. The commonest cause of red, swollen joints which first give trouble after age 40 is gout. The main tip-off to the early stages of this condition is that the joints become severely inflamed, often in the middle of the night, but usually subside completely without residual stiffness after a few days or weeks. Gout often occurs in people who are not addicted to high living. It affects the joint at the base of the toe, which most people think is typical of the disease, less than one fifth of the time. A *low purine diet* helps a great deal. Omit organ meats like sweetbreads and liver, navy and similar type beans, and soups or gravies. If you suspect gout, or if these foods make your joint trouble worse, check with your doctor for a more thorough diet and for special medicines if required.

Bodily rest. You can build your recuperative powers to fight arthritis with extra rest. Several breaks during the day are always helpful. More complete bed rest usually helps if you have fever weakness, or widespread involvement.

Rest for sore joints. Using red, swollen joints does much more harm than good, even though you definitely need the courage to use parts in spite of some discomfort when they are mildly involved or have begun to mend. If a joint becomes stiff and sore after a certain amount of use, or if it stiffens up 6 to 12 hours later, you should do somewhat less next time.

Motion-preserving exercises. You can cut your chance of later stiffness or crippling quite substantially by carrying each swollen joint through its entire range of motion several times a day. Do this immediately after or toward the end of the warm flannel treatment. If the involved joint is a· hinge, like a finger joint, elbow or knee, move it all the way one way then the other. More complex joints call for several varieties of loosening movement: you want to free up a sore shoulder so that you can raise your arm, move it forward and back, and rotate it, for instance.

Supported or flotation exercises. Some patients find that they do better with motion-preserving exercises if the weight of the moving part is supported. You can exercise under water in a warm tub, so that the part floats virtually weightless. You can support ailing parts with healthy ones, or get someone to help you. Do not force the part beyond where you can move it with its own muscles, though. Just relieve the burden imposed by the weight of the moving part.

Cripple-cutting braces. Even total loss of function in a joint usually involves very little crippling or disability if the joint freezes in a highly usable position. If you have a prolonged bout with joint trouble, make sure that the parts involved stay useful by bracing them in a workable position during your hours of rest. Follow these suggestions according to the parts involved:

Back: Sleep on a firm surface as described on page 20. Sleep on your back with a small pillow or rolled blanket between your shoulder blades so that the weight of your shoulders will keep them square. Place sandbags (made at home from light canvas) along both sides of your body so that you will not roll over during the night. Place a small pillow under your neck if necessary for comfort, but never place a pillow under your head.

Hips: Keep the legs from rolling outward by laying sandbags along the outside of your thigh and leg. Your toes should point straight up when you are in bed.

Knees: Lay sandbags along the sides of your legs to keep them straight so that the weight of your leg straightens your knees. If any stiffness develops, your legs will then remain entirely usable. Arthritics who sleep with their legs bent or with pillows under their knees sometimes find themselves in a crippling half-stoop if joints freeze up even slightly.

Ankles, feet, and toes: A footboard saves lots of crippling here! Cut a board 18 inches wide, one inch thick and four inches shorter than the width of your bed. Nail short crosspieces at right angles extending toward the head of the bed, to fit beneath the mattress and hold the footboard in perpendicular position. Place the footboard inside the top sheet when you make the bed. Keep your feet against it as you sleep to hold your ankles at the proper right angle and keep the weight of the covers from twisting inflamed toes.

Shoulders: Sleep with a pillow or sandbag between your elbow and your body to assure proper spacing.

Elbows: Keep your elbows partly bent, either by placing sandbags under them and laying your hands across your body or by raising your hands and forearms on two pillows. Even a totally stiff elbow is less of a handicap if you can still get your hand to your mouth and comb your hair.

Wrists: If your hand is tipped up at the wrist, you can use your finger muscles much more strongly than if the wrist is bent. A leather-padded metal splint helps to hold your hand up during the night. Buy one from the nearest surgical supply house, or have your shoemaker make a brace which fits from your palm to your midforearm. As a temporary measure, you can wrap the hand and wrist with an elastic bandage each night. With the wrist tipped up and the bandage partially stretched, wrap alternate turns around the wrist and around the hand at the base of the fingers, crossing at the back of the wrist or hand.

Subsiding or smoldering joint trouble: Home treatment really comes into its own in smoldering or subsiding joint troubles. You can't always afford a doctor for dragged-out complaints, and these difficulties yield especially well to remedies you can manage for yourself. Use full hormone-spurring doses of aspirin without fear, and take these additional measures:

Sore, stiff fingers yield very well to paraffin dip baths. Melt and cool paraffin-oil mixture as described on page 21. After testing the temperature, dip your better hand quickly in the paraffin. As soon as the first layer is set, dip again. Repeat until the paraffin forms a glove ¼ inch or more in thickness. Wrap in a dry towel to hold the heat. Now dip your worse hand in the mixture several times, letting each layer set before dipping again. When the paraffin forms a ¼ inch glove, immerse the whole hand in the melted paraffin and hold it there. The soothing warmth will penetrate all the way through your fingers in twenty to thirty minutes.

Joggers' knee. Actually, jogging shouldn't strain the knees any more than walking the same distance, if as much. If you jog with proper body mechanics, so that you land smoothly on the ball of your foot instead of on your heel, the shock of your knee at each stride is cushioned by the muscles of your calf. But most of the people who complain of jogger's knees would never walk as many miles a week as they jog, and the thousands of extra impacts involved cause them a good bit of discomfort.

The first point to check if you have knee discomfort after jogging is the straightness of your legs. Bow legs or knock knees place a great burden on knee ligaments while you jog. If you suffer from one of these conditions, it is better to switch to swimming or bicycling instead of jogging.

Mild joint inflammation from jogging responds to hot wet towels and aspirin or Tylenol. A whirlpool or shower massage also gives relief. If you continue to have trouble, special jogging shoes with a thick padded sole, fitted large enough to let you wear two pairs of athletic socks, may cut down the pounding. And ask the track coach at the nearest high school to watch you in action once—he may give you some tips on improved running technique to substantially reduce joint strain.

Aching arms, hips, or knees. Painted on paraffin does wonders here. Prepare the paraffin, then paint it on with a paint brush in layers until it is at least ¼ inch thick. Wrap with a dry towel to hold the heat. Peel off after thirty minutes, and follow with a rubdown using this homemade liniment:

Methyl salicylate (wintergreen)	¼ cup
Camphor and soap liniment	¾ cup

You can get these ingredients in any drug store, and mix them together in a clean, stoppered bottle. Shake well before each use. Rub in around the aching joint for 10 to 15 minutes.

Perpetual stiff neck. Make yourself a neck-stretching sling, as described on page 24. While your neck is under moderate stretch, turn your head far to the right. Place the heel of your right hand against the left side of your chin and gently press straight back. Repeat, turning your head to the left. Do this three times on each of three occasions through the day.

Stiff elbows, wrists, ankles, and toes. Use contrast baths for these forms of misery, following the directions on page 29. Paraffin baths help, too.

Tennis elbow. The athletic craze has hit as hard or harder in Minnesota than in the rest of the country. The lakeside paths teem with joggers, bicyclers and skaters, the tennis courts jam up at dawn and often remain in use far into the night (with the aid of floodlights). Even the living rooms of sedate older couples often sport an exercycle in front of the TV, where Dad or Mom pedals away while watching the news. And more power to them! On balance the exercise does much more good than harm (I'm something of an elderly jock myself). But all this exercise has led to a considerable fallout of muscle and joint miseries, the most prominent of which is tennis elbow. The exercise from which this unhappy condition stems might not always be tennis: I've seen "tennis elbow" after everything from too much golf to chopping wood or wielding a screwdriver. But the misery is always pretty much the same. Pain centers in the muscles at the front of the forearm just below the elbow and becomes intense with such motions as a firm handshake or an attempt to open a tight jar lid. The elbow usually won't go quite all the way straight, and carrying a briefcase or a bucket—anything which stretches the elbow toward straightness by passive pull—usually makes the condition much worse. Without treatment, it drags on for months and limits your activities severely.

During the early, acutely tender stage, the best treatment for tennis elbow is the same as described above for an inflamed joint: aspirin, contrast baths, rest (perhaps reinforced with an elastic bandage) and, in particular, avoidance of the twisting or stretching strains which make it hurt worse. As soon as the acute tenderness subsides, though, you can speed healing tremendously with a special exercise. Hold the arm as straight as it will go with your fingers and thumb extended. Turn your thumb as far as it will go toward the outside. With the arm still fully extended and turned, press upward on the bottom edge of a table or similar surface as hard as you can for five seconds or so. Relax for a few seconds and repeat four or five times. At first you will find this exercise quite uncomfortable, but *if done at full stretch* it will not aggravate the condition. As the muscle strengthens, the tennis elbow will disappear, usually within a week.

To avoid recurrence, continue the exercise once a day. If the aggravating factor was actually tennis, you can also help to avoid further trouble by shifting your grip. Most people who have tennis elbow hold the racquet so that it makes a considerable angle with their forearm. If you hold the racquet in this position and press the front of its far end against an unyielding surface, you will feel the strain on your rotator muscles—the ones affected by tennis elbow. Shift your grip so that the racquet runs diagonally along your hand and its shaft is directly in line with your forearm, then press the tip against an unyielding surface, and you will find that an entirely different set of muscles comes into use. You may need a slightly smaller racquet handle to make this work for you, but a shift in grip often works wonders in relieving strain.

Golfers and others can make similar changes in grip or stance to relieve rotator strain. And many other miseries caused by repetitive strain yield to the "exercise under full stretch" approach, from jogger's ankle to shoveler's shoulder. Locate the sore muscle, find a position which puts it under full stretch and exercise by isometric push. You'll find this technique helpful in many of the miseries induced by "overdoing it" in almost any sport or vigorous pursuit.

Diffuse joint trouble. When a patient tells me that he aches all over or points to half a dozen different ailing joints, I usually ask him to build himself a baker. The essential features are several light bulbs and sockets, a reflecting surface of metal or foil, and a frame which holds the light bulbs with the reflector about 18 inches away from the painful body parts. Most patients make a rod iron and sheet tin or aluminum structure in the shape of a tunnel (as one of the two parts of a cylinder cut in half along its length), then fasten two to four sockets to its under surface for a bank of 100- to 200-watt light bulbs. The heat from light bulbs in such a unit is very soothing and much more even than that you get from a heating pad or single-unit heat lamp. You can lie with your sore joints underneath the baker for 30 to 45 minutes once or twice each day.

Home whirlpool equipment. Although the equipment is rather expensive, several of my patients have reported worthwhile relief from home whirlpool treatments. A special pump swirls the water in your bathtub around and fills it with tiny air bubbles. The effect is of combined heat and massage, easily applied without assistance to almost any body part. The outfit my patients use is made by Jacuzzi Bros. Inc. here in Minneapolis, but there may be others just as good. I wouldn't try to improvise a homemade substitute because of the danger of electric equipment around bathroom fixtures. For red or swollen joints, only moderately warm water (about 108° F.) works best. Smoldering miseries may respond to somewhat warmer temperatures (about 112° F.).

Hip, knee, and joint strain. You can avoid or relieve a great deal of joint distress by controlling strain in weight-bearing joints. These joints can usually bear up under their share of your normal weight. But an overloaded joint is like a tire on a car that's loaded until the wheels scrape the fenders. A little extra weight causes a lot of extra strain, wear, and tear.

Aching knees, for instance, are often due to extra strain produced when flat feet shift the muscle pulls in the leg. In other cases, undue strain on the knees stems from knock-knees or bow-legs. You can relieve most such undue strain in a hurry with inconspicuous shoe wedges that rebalance your weight. Here's the step-by-step program:

1. Get a pair of oxford style shoes, with at least four eyelets for laces on each side and with low heels.

2. Unless the heels fit so snugly that your feet will not roll inside the shoes even a fraction of an inch, get your shoemaker to make molded heel counters (cost: about $4.00).

3. Have half inch heel wedges put on for another dollar or two to tip your feet as follows: for flat feet or knock knees, have wedges installed on the *inside* of your heels, shifting extra weight to the outer, little-toe side of your foot. For bow legs, have wedges installed on the *outside* of your heels to shift extra weight to the arched side of your foot (but fit arch supports at

the same time if your feet are the least bit weak—this position puts extra stress on the arches).

You can also relieve joint strain by shedding excess weight. Aching ankles, knees, and hips do better without the burden of extra pounds. Even a few pounds of weight loss often gives striking relief.

Growing pains. Minnesota brings out the vigor of the young. It's not just the great chances for outdoor activities—other places have toboggan slopes, ice rinks, and shovelable walks. It's the confounded cold, which keeps you going at full steam just to keep warm.

But youngsters in other regions aren't too much different. They race around at full speed, keep going until they're exhausted, and ignore the rough ground or poor footing. No wonder they get aches and pains occasionally! If you or I tried to keep up with one of them, we'd wind up sick in bed.

So they complain of muscle aches, joint pains, "stitches" (which are side aches caused by muscle spasm in the diaphragm), and so forth. Mainly your problem isn't what to do about these complaints—youngsters mend quickly, and the pains are often gone before you can get a boy or girl to hold still for warm soaks or swallow an aspirin. The problem is that "growing pains" sometimes turn out to be early evidence of rheumatic fever. Prompt identification and care for this disorder generally helps the victim to avoid heart involvement, so it pays to lean over backward in checking out any truly suspicious complaints.

The simplest checkup is still with the old thermometer. When a youngster complains of growing pains, your first step should be to take his temperature three times a day, in the morning, right after school and at bedtime. Shake the thermometer all the way down and be sure that it has registered completely (by reading it quickly, putting it back in the mouth for a while and reading it again until it stays the same). Sometimes you'll find a mildly elevated temperature in the afternoon when you hadn't noted fever. More important, you'll sometimes find a variation of more than one full degree between morning and evening readings. Even if none of the readings go over 98.6 degrees, more than a one degree low-high spread makes rheumatic fever a distinct possibility.

Finally, you can check for extra warmth or heat in the area of each complaint, especially if a joint is involved. Feel for temperature change with the back of your fingers or hand rather than with the palm (which is more sensitive to touch but less sensitive to warmth and cold). Compare the part that hurts with the opposite member, and if there is any trace of extra warmth, arrange for a checkup with your doctor.

HOME REMEDIES FOR NEURITIS, BURSITIS, AND INFLAMED LEADER GUIDES

A great many of the miseries that go with rheumatism stem from other structures than the joints themselves. Some of these troubles come on with joint difficulty, others strike independently. Home measures help a great deal, with little or no expense.

Neuritis and neuralgia. If you tend toward joint trouble, you usually also suffer at times from shooting pains, numbness, tingling or supersensitive skin. Three measures help these complaints:

Vitamin B1. Vitamin B1 (*thiamine*) seems to speed healing of neuritis and neuralgia. Two 50 mgm. tablets a day is an average effective intake.

Massage with homemade wintergreen liniments. For this kind of discomfort, mix:

Methyl salicylate (oil of wintergreen)	½ cup
Camphor and soap liniment	½ cup

Rub in with long, even strokes for 10 to 15 minutes three times daily.

Flannel or cotton knit protection. The gentle softness and warmth of flannel wrapping or cotton knit long underwear proves very soothing to neuritis and neuralgia. Such dressing also prevents the discomfort caused by rubbing of harsher fabrics on raw-nerve sensitive skin.

Bursitis. Bursitis usually involves a shoulder, elbow, or knee. In these locations, muscles and tendons glide across each other or rub along bony prominences. Your body forms smooth-lined pockets of tissue to ease the friction. When these bearing-sacs get sore, the scraping of raw, sensitive surfaces gives exquisite pain.

If you get severe bursitis, your doctor can give worthwhile help. Hydrocortisone injections, X-ray treatment and several other measures are very effective. With milder attacks, these four simple home remedies may do the trick:

Pressure bandaging. An elastic bandage wrapped snugly around the area involved often braces the inflamed bursa. You can usually wrap the area near a joint comfortably with Figure 8 loops—a turn above the joint, a diagonal turn down across it, a turn below the joint and a diagonal back up. Keep the bandage partly stretched as you apply it. If the bursa is very tender, wind on several strips of soft flannel before using the elastic bandage.

Lightbulb heat. Since the area involved in bursitis is usually fairly small, lightbulb heat from an ordinary desk lamp usually gives considerable relief. Place the bulb 12 to 18 inches from your bared skin. If you do not have a desk lamp or metal reflector, line a cloth shade with aluminum foil to help reflect and concentrate the heat.

Hormone-boosting doses of aspirin. For quick relief from bursitis, take aspirin in the dosage and with the precautions described on page 48. Continue half doses for at least a week after the disorder begins to subside.

Rest. Occasionally, the only way to get relief from bursitis is to keep from using the affected part for a few days. If an arm or shoulder is involved, a sling usually helps. In other parts, deliberately sparing the sore part pays. Remember that bursitis pain comes from rubbing raw surfaces together, and this rubbing itself makes the surfaces rawer still.

Leader guide inflammation. The commonest form of this complaint is excruciating soreness and swelling of the forearm when you have done a job which requires repeatedly making the same motion with your hand or wrist, like painting or driving nails. If you lay your other hand on the sore wrist, you may be able to feel a creaking like that of a leather saddle. Inflammation of the leaders' lubricated sheaths may strike in the hand or ankle, too. These miseries drag on and on unless you use intensive treatment, but they respond very well to these home measures:

Aspirin in the doses described above helps to keep you comfortable and to speed healing.

Splinting is absolutely necessary, and must extend to all of the parts which can be moved by the sore muscles. Tendon sheath inflammation in the wrist calls for bandaging the whole hand and wrist, for instance. I generally pad a light piece of board well and bind it to the top of the fingers, wrist and forearm with an elastic bandage.

Contrast baths three or four times a day are well worth the effort. See page 29 for specific directions.

4

How to Prevail Over
Constipation

If constipation has never plagued you, you have been fortunate indeed. Most people need to give definite attention to their bowel function at fairly frequent intervals, if not continually. Yet you can almost always control constipation completely with home measures. By steering clear of the easy but temporary means of relief, you can correct constipation without irritating your bowel and perpetuating your difficulty. Throw your convenient but ultimately harmful laxative pills out the window and try this effective, step-by-step program for total correction of a tight bowel.

STEP-BY-STEP CORRECTION OF TIGHT BOWELS

Step One: Give your bowel a rest on a low-bulk diet. Your bowel has probably been irritated by laxatives, overworked by bulk-formers, or scraped insensitive by dry bulk passages. Let it rest and heal itself for about two weeks before trying to achieve unaided, comfortably regular movements. A low-bulk diet provides the rest phase of your constipation cure. You can eat freely of meat, dairy products, eggs, and bread. Eat two normal servings of fruit or juice a day, one of lemon, orange, or grapefruit and one of bananas, pears, peaches, peeled apricots, baked apple, or strawberries. Also eat two servings of well-cooked peas, string beans, carrots, beets, spinach, tomato or potato, and avoid caffeine.

During this time, you should take a *salt and soda enema* whenever you have discomforts like headache, nausea and cramps, or whenever you go more than three days without a movement. Follow this technique for a comfortable effective enema:

Dissolve one teaspoonful of table salt and two teaspoonfuls of baking soda in one quart of lukewarm water. Place in an enema bag. Use the smallest enema tip. Lubricate well with petroleum jelly. Lie on your left side, and insert the tip just far enough that it stays. Gradually raise the enema bag until it is one to two feet above the level of the enema tip, and let the mixture flow in gently. If abdominal discomfort develops, lower the bag somewhat and gently knead the left lower portion of your abdomen with your free hand. When the enema has all run in, remove the tip and prepare for an evacuation. As soon as an urge develops, the enema is working fully: you need not try to hold back.

Some patients find that somewhat larger enemas are perfectly comfortable and extra effective. If you feel that evacuations produced by one quart enemas are not adequate, put double quantities in the enema bag and run in as much as you can comfortably absorb.

On the other hand, if full-sized enemas cause too much discomfort or if your circumstances (such as often being away from home overnight) make them inconvenient, a Fleet's Disposable Enema Kit or a similar product is available without a prescription in any drugstore at modest cost. A special concentration of salt substances makes a few ounces of solution do a good job for most victims of constipation, and the outfit (with a plastic squeeze bottle and ready-lubricated tip) is completely ready to use.

If movements have been hard and massive, you can ease their passage with *preliminary internal oiling*. Place two ounces of warm olive oil into the rectum with a rubber ear or infant syringe half an hour or more before preparing the salt and soda solution or using Fleet's Kit.

Step Two: Gradually increase moist-bulk foods. When you have achieved a rested, irritation-free bowel, your next step is to increase gradually the amount of *moist-bulk producing* fruit you eat each day. Milder, never-irritating fruits should be chosen first. These are stewed prunes, cantaloupe or honeydew melon, raisins, currants, applesauce, plums, cherries and berries. More irritating fruits like figs and dates are often very helpful, but must be tried at first with caution. If you have a sensitive bowel, they may do more harm than good. Raw apples must also be used with caution: they often cause gas in the presence of sluggish bile flow or gall bladder trouble.

During the moist-bulk increasing phase, most sufferers find that they need a little *mild lubricating or moisturizing medicine* for their bowel. A tablespoonful twice a day of any mineral oil emulsion like Petrolagar or Petromul does the trick. Be sure you use the plain emulsion, without added phenolphthalein or cascara. Moisture-holding colloids like Mucilose or Metamucil and stool softeners such as Surfak also do an excellent job. Take one heaping teaspoonful in a glass of water morning and evening at first, following each dose with a full glass of water. A higher or lower dose may work better for you, but wait several days before deciding what you need.

Meanwhile, use enemas if you get very uncomfortable. The dose can be cut down gradually over a period of weeks as natural moist-bulk foods take over your body's requirements.

If abdominal comfort and easily-passed stools cannot be achieved by these means, you probably need *spasm-relaxing medicines* or other special measures. Doan's "kidney pills" (which contain spasm-soothing Hyoscine), Donnatal liquid, or Wyanoids suppositories will give some benefit, until you can get your doctor to prescribe stronger tablets or liquids. But remember that your aim is comfort, not stools of a certain size or frequency. Most people who fail at this point get discouraged because they have small, infrequent stools—a natural effect of low-bulk eating. Forget false notions about needing a bowel movement every day or every two days. The key to a better-working bowel is regulation that fits in with *your* body's natural patterns without nausea, headache, bloating, cramps, or difficult-to-pass, hard stools. Even if your natural rhythm proves to produce only one movement a week, you should be content so long as that movement is normally sausage-shaped and you do not suffer gas pains beforehand.

Step Three: Free yourself gradually of all bowel-regulating medicines. Medicines are only a crutch to keep you comfortable until new mental, physical, and food habits solve your bowel problem. However, any abrupt change may throw your bowel out of kilter. Medicines should be tapered slowly, taking a dose every single day, but decreasing the dose very gradually over a period of six to eight weeks. You may need an occasional enema during this time if you cut down your medicine too quickly. Don't be discouraged. If you taper slowly enough you will almost always ultimately get along without any medicines at all, and with very infrequent enemas.

How Mrs. Jacob followed the three steps to natural rhythm regulation. Mrs. Jacob had taken laxatives every two or three days for more than twenty years.

"Lots of doctors have told me to quit laxatives," she told me. "But if I don't take something, I get miserable. Headache, gas pains, upset stomach—it's more than I can bear."

Mrs. Jacob followed the three step program we've just discussed. When she set her bowel at rest with a low bulk diet and enemas, she remained entirely comfortable. During Step Two she took a full tablespoonful of Metamucil twice a day at first, and tapered very slowly. She got used to eating fruit with each meal, and drinking plenty of water. At the end of four months, she was freed forever of the need for laxatives, and settled into a regular, comfortable bowel rhythm with two or three movements a week.

CONSTIPATION IN CHILDREN

When a mother brings a child into my office with the complaint of constipation, the first thing I want to know is whether the *child* complained or whether the nature and frequency of movements upset the *mother*. Infrequent movements alone don't upset *me*. Stomach aches or loss of appetite (with or without constipation) make me want to check a stool specimen for worm eggs before I treat bowel rhythm. After sorting out these separate problems, though, I still find quite a few youngsters with constipation.

The toughest job we adults have with these youngsters is convincing them that cola drinks and candy don't "make it." Colas contain just as much caffeine as coffee, and have two harmful effects. Caffeine often throws the bowel into spasm and causes constipation. It always increases the flow of fluid through your kidneys and dries out your system instead of supplying needed internal moisture. Candy creates problems in a different way—not for what it is, but for what it replaces. Every candy bar kills the appetite as thoroughly as two or three pieces of fruit, for instance, and provides neither bulk nor moisture. It's hard to make these points without sounding like an old fogy, but maybe you can accomplish at least something by making your household purchases according to these rules. If youngsters get ginger ale and fresh fruit out of the refrigerator for nothing, maybe they'll spend a little less of their "own money" on the less desirable alternatives.

Parents often have difficulty getting themselves to give their children an enema. It may be easier to spread some newspaper or other padding on the bathroom floor to administer the solution than it is to transport the child from the bedroom after giving the solution. Youngsters below age twelve do well with a pint of salt and soda solution (half quantities of each ingredient) or with a child's size Fleet's Enema. The former has the advantage that it can be expelled immediately, while the disposable kit solution has to be retained 5 minutes. In smaller children, glycerine suppositories (obtainable without a prescription) often give temporary relief just as effectively as an enema with a lot less bother. Keep these in the refrigerator or else they get too soft to insert readily. Unwrap and insert blunt-end first, then get the child to hold the suppository in for five minutes or so.

Infants need formula change for constipation, so you should call your doctor.

HOW TO FIGHT THE NATURAL TENDENCY
TOWARD CONSTIPATION

Even if constipation has never plagued you enough to require a full-scale program for correction, you will probably find that measures to avoid it are worthwhile at times. Several techniques are easy to work into your daily way of life without consuming extra time, effort or money:

How to empty your lower bowel efficiently. You may make bowel movements much easier by following these simple toileting rules:

Take plenty of time, at the same time every day. After breakfast, or whenever you find movements most frequent, set aside 10 or 15 minutes for elimination. At first you may rarely have movements at this time. But if you persist, your body will train itself to take advantage of the opportunity.

Read, listen to a portable radio, or relax mentally during toileting. Worry and tension clamp down your bowel into a stiff, inactive tube. Keep yourself distracted from concerns of the past or future while you're encouraging nature's call.

Flexed hips help your belly muscles work better at the toilet; a 6″ or 8″ footstool under your feet often makes elimination much easier.

Exercise. Your abdominal muscles, contracting in the course of everyday activity, massage the bowel. This massage helps to move bowel contents along until they can be eliminated. If you walk 10 to 20 blocks each day, the resulting muscular action makes your bowels move more freely.

Abdominal massage. If you do not have time to exercise, you can easily use your hands to replace muscular massage as follows:

Lie down and let your abdominal muscles go entirely loose. Place your right hand on the lowest part of the abdomen to the right of center. Press the little finger side firmly down and into the abdomen. Roll your hand slowly toward the thumb side, as if you were kneading margarine along inside a sack. Place your left hand adjoining. Press the little finger side in, then roll toward the thumb side. Massage in this fashion up the right side of the abdomen, across the upper part, and down the left side. Then begin again low on the right. Continue massage for about five minutes.

Dodge dry bulk. Moist-bulk foods have always been the constipation victim's first standby. Fruits and cooked vegetables add moisture-holding bulk, and extra moisture makes movements easier. But it's the moisture that does the trick, not the bulk. Extra bulk in any form means extra work for your bowel, and dry bulk means extra work without extra moisture or other benefit.

Any victim of constipation should avoid these dry-bulk forming foods like the plague:

> Raw vegetables, especially rabbit-food type salads.
> Cabbage, brussels sprouts, and broccoli.
> Bran cereals.

Less tension means less constipation. Another effective way to fend off constipation is to relieve the tension which so often brings it on.

"When my wife helps me pack," one traveling man told me, "she'll stand there with my bottle of laxative pills and say: 'Is this trip going to be a chore or a pleasure?' If I say chore, she throws them in. If it's pleasure I never have the need."

If you control or air tensions you'll have much less trouble with constipation. You *can* control tension, usually without the aid of drugs or medicines. Simple home measures can help greatly in bringing tranquil calmness to your daily life.

How to hold up better under tension. You'll find that one controllable human trait adds greatly to tension: trying to grapple with the past or future in some corner of your mind at the same time that you attack the problems or manage the tasks of the present moment. While you cook the supper, you try to figure what you should have said in yesterday's argument, or you try to plan tomorrow's meals. While you do your job, you try to figure out how you got so far behind on your bills or what to get your wife for Christmas. The human mind is not meant to grapple with the separate problems of the past, the present, and the future at one time.

You can worry less and accomplish more if you take up problems one at a time. Live right now. Occupy your mind by chatting with your husband, listening to the radio, or adding other pleasant stimulations to the present moment. Then take time out: forget about right now and plan for later. Grapple with the present and the future separately instead of both at once, and forget most problems from the past.

TEMPORARY RELIEF WITHOUT LONG-RANGE HARM

If your bowel gets tight, you need relief. Most ordinary laxatives lead you into a vicious circle, though. They give temporary relief, but they irritate the lining of your bowel sufficiently that further tightness often develops. You can often keep yourself from getting into a really prolonged bout with constipation simply by sticking to these measures for temporary relief:

Enemas. A salt and soda enema, given according to the directions above, will never cause further bowel irritation or self-perpetuating constipation. Use enemas as often as necessary for relief of sporadic episodes.

Disposable enema kits. If you are traveling or otherwise unable to use standard enema technique, the Fleet's disposable plastic enema outfit works very comfortably and efficiently. By using a special concentrated solution, this outfit gives as much relief from a cupful of material as you would otherwise get from a quart.

Phosphates. If any form of enema is absolutely impractical, an occasional dose of Fleet's Phospho-Soda is probably the most harmless and convenient means of ready relief. One or two teaspoonfuls in a half a glassful of water before breakfast usually give relief by ten a.m. This material has the one drawback that its demands are rather urgent when they arise, so you should not stray too far from facilities.

Rid yourself of constipation worries. Constipation worries are plagues in themselves. Whether you take action against sluggish bowel function or not, take heart from these reassuring facts:

> You do not soak up poisons from inside a sluggish bowel. Headache, gas pains, nausea, and other constipation-caused complaints come from pressure on sensitive nerve endings in the rectum. People subject to these complaints are made just as miserable by a rectum packed with cotton as by actual bowel stagnation.

> You do not need a movement every day or every other day. Some people average only one movement a week, and still enjoy quiet, comfortable abdomens and soft, easily passed stools. Strive for natural rhythm regulation with good bowel action at your body's own, individually determined interval. Don't try to put your bowel in a time-interval strait jacket.

> Small movements may be completely adequate. If a movement passes easily, is of normal consistency, and is not rushed or interrupted, you need not worry about whether it is large enough or not.

> Intestinal fermentation simply does not occur. Most stomach and intestinal gas comes from swallowed air. Poisonous gases do not form even if material moves through the intestine very slowly.

SPECIAL FORMS OF CONSTIPATION

A tight bowel occasionally springs from more serious causes than ordinary constipation. Sometimes victims of more serious types can get considerable help from home remedies. On other occasions, their awareness of what is going on may lead to better results through prompt doctor care.

Rectal accumulations. An uncomfortable plug of hardened material sometimes accumulates in the rectum. People over sixty who are physically inactive often suffer from this condition. You can usually tell that a plug is accumulating, but straining produces only a little watery discharge. Ordinary enemas give no relief. Severe lower abdominal cramps frequently follow, with loss of appetite, nausea, and sometimes headache.

Oil enemas. You can often get rid of rectal accumulations with simple home measures. The first thing to try is a *slow-action oil enema*. At bedtime, place one cup of warm olive oil in an ordinary enema bag. Use the smallest available tip, and lubricate it well with petroleum jelly. Lie on your left side. Let the oil run in very slowly. Keep your abdomen relaxed. Stop the flow and take several deep breaths through your mouth if you get an urge to expel the oil. When all the oil has run in, withdraw the tip. Lie flat on your back with your buttocks pressed together until you have no further urge to expel the oil, then let it soak in overnight. In the morning, a gentle evacuation often occurs after breakfast. If not, a salt and soda enema is often more effective and more comfortable than it would have been without the oil.

Blocked bowel. Blocked bowel always arises out of some other condition. The vanguards of blocked bowel usually give considerable warning. You can make their cure safer and more comfortable if you get help with them before the final blockage occurs.

Hernia is the commonest cause of blocked bowel. It also gives the longest and most easily detected warning. In hernia, organs which belong inside the abdomen slide through a narrow opening in the abdomen's muscle sheath. This happens most commonly in the groin. Sometimes it occurs at or above the navel or within the scar left by a previous operation. If you get a hernia, you will notice a bulging under the skin which shows up more when you strain at stool, or cough. You will not usually have pain, although the stretched muscles in the area may become stiff and sore after you have done heavy work. You may get a sliding or pulling sensation when you cough or strain.

A hernia is dangerous because a length of bowel can slide into it and get stuck. The narrow gap in muscle through which the hernia slides can act just like a noose around your intestine, blocking off the movement of bowel contents. Intestinal obstruction leads to severe cramps all over the abdomen, vomiting, shock, and truly grave illness. If you have any signs of hernia, ward off blocked bowel by seeing your doctor and following his advice. That advice will probably include an operation, but a safe, relatively comfortable one compared with the risks you'll avoid.

The most important other cause of blocked bowel is tumor. A tumor also gives warning, but in less definite ways. Although innocent conditions might well be at fault, you should see your doctor whenever you note any of these signs:

1. Indigestion over a period of three weeks or more.
2. Unexplained weight loss.
3. Abruptly beginning constipation, diarrhea or alternate spells of constipation and diarrhea.
4. Frequent feeling that bowels need to move when an attempt to do so proves futile.

How Harvey Peterson beat his tumor to the punch. When tumor singles out a victim, that person still can win his way back to perfect health. Harvey Peterson's case is a good example. When Harvey first came to my office, he said:

"I've been constipated for the first time in my life these last six weeks. And this morning there was a little blood with my movement. Probably nothing serious, but when you're over forty I guess you can't afford to wait and see."

It's a good thing Harvey felt that way. About a foot from the lower end of his bowel, a tumor surrounded his intestine in a tight, hard band. In a few more weeks or months, that tumor would have blocked the bowel completely, causing painful and dangerous obstruction. But Harvey never suffered that dread state. He had an operation, but not a hurried or extra-hazardous one. Harvey was out of the hospital in ten days and back at work in a month, completely and permanently cured of his disease.

5

How to Fight Diarrhea, Indigestion, Stomach Ulcers, and Gall Bladder Trouble

You seldom hear a North Country citizen complain of diarrhea or stomach upset, but the reason is a trick of language, not an iron-clad intestine. Any brief difficulty with the stomach or bowels is "stomach flu" to a Minnesotan. In spite of a phlegmatic temperament and uniformly clean kitchens, our Scandinavian and Deutschlander citizens have had lots of chance to try home remedies against indigestion and diarrhea. Instead of ignoring such discomfort until it goes away or taking some remedy you have seen advertised on TV, why don't you try the effective steps they have worked out over the years?

HOME REMEDIES FOR DIARRHEA

The outlander blames our smorgasbord, the native blames outlander's germs, but they both suffer the same miseries and need the same measures for relief when diarrhea strikes. Home treatment is often highly effective for loose or watery bowel movements, and is perfectly safe for any adult to try so long as there is no evidence of serious disease (such as pain which might be due to appendicitis).

The long fast. The most effective single method you can use to stop an attack of diarrhea is a period of absolute fasting. Whenever nausea or severe loss of appetite accompanies diarrhea, you will do better to omit even water the first six to twelve hours. If your stomach seems unaffected, you can take water, strained fruit juice, ginger ale, weak tea or clear broth. Moderately cooled beverages and lukewarm soup cause less cramps or upset than ice cold or hot liquids. You will find that very small quantities at frequent intervals sit better than a whole glassful or bowl at a time.

Bowel-flushing enemas. Strange as it seems, an enema often gives you a lot of relief and speeds your recovery from diarrhea. The germs that underlie most attacks actually die out very quickly, but the poisons they leave behind continue to irritate the bowel lining for some time. A thorough cleansing enema rids you of those poisons much more quickly and comfortably than more watery movements. One formula that usually does the job without stirring up hardly any cramping or discomfort is this:

Table salt	1 teaspoonful
Baking soda	2 teaspoonfuls
Warm water	1 quart

Use a small tip, well lubricated with petroleum jelly. Lie on your left side. Let the fluid run in slowly. Whenever you feel uncomfortably full or get any trace of a cramp, stop the flow, take several deep breaths and knead deeply but gently along the left side of your abdomen from below upward with the flat of your fingers. When the enema is complete, or when you find that further flow makes uncomfortable pressure even after a two minute rest with massage, you may expel it immediately. There is no need to hold in the solution to get full effect.

Most ordinary episodes of diarrhea respond to a single, thorough cleansing enema. In very severe attacks, two or three enemas at intervals of one to four hours may be needed. You can use cleansing enemas as often as recurrence of diarrhea and griping shows the need.

Fluid restoring enemas. The dragged-out feeling and fever which often accompany diarrhea stem partly from loss of body fluid. Watery stools can make diarrhea a serious illness even in adults, especially if nausea or vomiting keeps you from drinking anything. When an attack of diarrhea first starts, you should weigh yourself on an accurate scale. If the attack is severe, weigh yourself again at intervals through the day. If you lose more than five pounds or more than three per cent of your body weight, try taking one to four ounces of lukewarm water as an enema every 30 to 60 minutes. Deliver the fluid slowly. Press the cheeks of your buttocks together with both hands and lie still with your legs straight for five minutes or so afterward. Your body will soak the liquid up quickly. If your weight drops 5 to 8 pounds or 5 per cent, your doctor can probably speed your recovery with injections of fluid or with other prescription measures.

Diarrhea in children. Fluid loss causes special problems in infants and young children. Perhaps the easiest way to explain the problem is to look at a pound of our good Minnesota butter. Leave that pound in one piece and it has six surfaces—four sides, a top and a bottom. Cut it in half and the surface area is substantially increased—both cut surfaces are now added to the area already exposed.

The smaller the object the greater its surface per pound. This is true both of butter and human beings. There's an additional complication with children, though, because this principle applies to all kinds of surfaces, not just to the body's outside. A baby has many times more gut lining area per pound than an adult, and more lung lining, and more skin. Since he can lose fluid from all of these surfaces, fever and diarrhea dry him out in a hurry.

The best way to judge a child's or baby's water loss is by abrupt weight change, but if you don't have a sufficiently accurate scale you can use the *skin snap-back test*. You might check your youngsters with this technique right now, so you'll recognize any change from their normal. Just pinch up a fold of loose skin on an arm or abdomen and watch how quickly it springs back into place. If springback becomes definitely sluggish during an attack of diarrhea, best call your doctor—fluid injections may save a lot of difficulty later. For borderline sluggishness in snapback, try fluid replacement enemas of half an ounce to an ounce delivered with an infant syringe very slowly, and with the child's buttocks held together for five minutes afterward to make release less likely. A really dry youngster can soak up fluid from the rectum faster than you would believe—half an ounce to an ounce every half hour or so if necessary, and every hour in almost every case. I've seen many situations in which this much extra fluid kept a child from getting into the dehydration-fever-more-dehydration circle and prevented need for hospital-type injection care.

Don't neglect cleansing type enemas with youngsters, either. Use the same proportions of salt and soda with smaller quantities—two ounces for infants and four to eight ounces for older children—or use Fleet's Disposable Enema Kits (ready mixed, in a disposable plastic squeeze bottle) which come in both children's and adult sizes and cost about a dollar at any drugstore.

Kaolin compounds. You can buy several preparations like Kaopectate or Pectocil which help to soak up poisons as they travel through the intestine. You will benefit from using a remedy of this type if your stomach is not too upset to permit it. However, the doses recommended on the bottle are almost always much too small. Pick a compound with no dangerous antispasmodics, the active ingredients being kaolin and pectin only, and take two tablespoonfuls at least four times a day for 24 to 48 hours.

Stepwise reintroduction of foods. About half the patients who come to me for diarrhea have already virtually cured themselves once, then brought back the problem by eating solid food too quickly. You can help to speed and maintain your recovery from diarrhea by following this schedule.

Take nothing to eat or drink until at least two hours after onset of the diarrhea, or until four hours after any nausea or vomiting has ceased.

Start on moderately cooled or room temperature ginger ale, either straight or mixed with a little fruit juice. Sip this slowly from a small juice glass, taking at least ten minutes to down the first small serving. If this causes no upset, wait half an hour to an hour, then try another small portion. Continue small servings of ginger ale, fruit juice, weak tea or clear broth at quarter hour intervals until the diarrhea has been stopped for at least six hours, which will usually be about twelve hours from the onset of the illness.

At this point, take custards, soft boiled or poached eggs, toast, cooked cereal, and bland soups like chicken noodle or chicken rice. Wait at least 24 hours before you eat ordinary food. If you get the least sign of nausea, diarrhea, or severe loss of appetite, quit food and liquid again for four to six hours and start back on liquids.

Salt. Watery stools wash a great deal of salt out of your system, with the result that you often feel weary and dragged out for days or weeks afterward. The best restorative for this post-diarrhea drag is plain table salt. Salt your foods heavily, put lots of salty meats and dishes on the menu. If you tire very, very easily, take heat-fatigue-type salt tablets three or four times a day for about a week.

Allergic diarrhea. If you have a food allergy, some ordinary foodstuffs which are completely harmless to other people may be digestive poisons to you. They almost always cause diarrhea, often with belching, gas pains, or vomiting. A tip-off to this condition is sometimes the undigested state of the food that passes: you may still be able to identify every item eaten. Another tip-off is that once the offending meal is gone the symptoms usually quit with no left-over weakness or loss of appetite. Most victims also have many relatives with hay fever, hives, asthma, or migraine. You'll find a full discussion of this problem in the new chapter on food allergies (Chapter 2).

HOW TO CONTROL DIGESTIVE DISTRESS

You can relieve most mild or sporadic digestive distress for yourself, without a doctor's care. Before you try home measures, though, you should always ask yourself two questions:

1. Could this attack be appendicitis? Cramps from appendicitis often start in the pit of your stomach. Although they usually settle into your right side, pain and soreness often center on the left or up fairly high in the abdomen. If any one area of your abdomen is particularly tender in conjunction with abdominal cramps and either with or without nausea, appendicitis could be at fault. Certainly, you should check with your doctor within six hours after abdominal pain starts if you have not been able to obtain complete relief, even if the situation seems to be getting better. Be particularly alert for appendicitis in older children. Youngsters between nine and fourteen know enough about appendicitis to conceal symptoms from their parents in an effort to avoid an operation, but not enough to realize the danger of this course.

2. Have attacks been sufficiently regular to suggest a serious underlying cause? Indigestion which occurs two or three times a week for three weeks or more deserves medical attention even if it is easy to control with home measures. Such attacks sometimes stem from serious ulcers, tumor, or other illnesses for which your doctor can give considerably more aid if he sees you before the disease gets a head start.

If you can answer both these questions with a ringing "No," home remedies are worth a thorough trial. The proper approach varies according to whether your main complaint is heartburn, sick stomach, or gas and pressure pains.

Heartburn. A burning sensation or hot lump in the pit of the stomach fifteen to sixty minutes after a meal usually yields to *antacids* like baking soda, milk of magnesia or aluminum hydroxide. If you take baking soda, use one teaspoonful in half a glass of water. After about half an hour, if your symptoms are fairly well relieved, take a cup of warm milk or chocolate to keep down acid rebound. Milk of magnesia or aluminum hydroxide does not always give quite as good relief from the initial attack, but causes no acid rebound. They work very well for mild or early attacks. If you take aluminum hydroxide tablets, be sure to chew them thoroughly and take at least half a glass of water with each pill.

Sick stomach. If your main complaint is nausea, the key point is what you *eat and drink.* A thorough rest for your stomach through complete fasting generally helps. After about six hours, you can start on ginger ale or mixtures of ginger ale and fruit juice, not too cold, or on clear, lukewarm broth. If this sits well, you can start cooked cereal, soup, poached or boiled eggs, and toast after another six hours. Usually, it is wise to avoid ketchup, mustard and other strong seasonings for three to five days. Straight liquor or cocktails may stir up trouble, too, although tall drinks or wine usually do not.

Sleeping tablets. One of the best medicines for sick stomach is ordinary sleeping tablets. If you have some of these on hand, the dose recommended for bedtime use will usually quell your nausea at the price of only slight drowsiness if you stay on your feet. Take no more than half doses if you plan to operate an automobile or any hazardous machinery, though.

Prescription nausea fighters. Compazine and Thorazine work wonders with nausea and vomiting. You'll have to get your doctor on the phone to okay their use, since they are sold on prescription only. He'll tell you about dosage (which varies with your weight) and choose the right form (which varies with the length of action required).

. If you have a lot of "24-hour stomach flu" around your area—brief attacks of vomiting without pain that sweep through the family—it's not a bad idea to get your doctor to okay a few Compazine suppositories for you to keep around the house. These allow you to follow the "complete rest for the system—nothing to eat or drink" rule and still get prompt medicinal relief. Just unwrap a suppository and insert it into the rectum blunt-end first. The medicine soaks in directly from your intestine, and usually controls nausea and vomiting within half an hour.

Gas and pressure pains. The best single measure here is a *carminative enema*. Be sure that no areas of tenderness or other signs of appendicitis or infection are present. Set up the enema bag and fill it with one quart of water at 115 degrees, which is about as hot as your fingers can stand. Add two teaspoonfuls of spirits of peppermint or tincture of asafetida. Allow the mixture to run in slowly, with pauses and deep breaths to allow griping or discomfort to subside. Try to retain this enema for three to five minutes, giving gentle kneading massage to the abdomen during this period.

In milder cases, or if there is any tenderness, a small *gas-moving enema* works better. This involves half a cup of warm water, a teaspoonful of glycerine, and a level tablespoonful of Epsom salts. Retain this enema for five to ten minutes if possible.

Suppositories. The highly effective spasm soothing ingredient of some hemorrhoidal suppositories makes them a good home substitute for prescription-only tablets and liquids. "Wyanoids" contain enough belladonna to soak in through the rectal lining and give relief throughout your entire intestinal tract. Insert one immediately after a carminative or gas-moving enema has been evacuated for extra prompt action.

Spasm soothers. Your doctor will probably be glad to have you keep some prescription-type spasm soothers on hand in your medicine chest once he has picked a preparation and dosage which is one hundred per cent safe for you. If you have frequent difficulties, ask him what he recommends for your type of attack the next time you visit his office.

Low residue diet. If less material has to pass on through your intestine, cramp-causing spasms are less likely to develop. The main sources of indigestible fiber are raw vegetables, including most salad greens, the cabbage family (cabbage, brussels sprouts, and broccoli) and bran cereals. You often get considerable relief from cramps by omitting these foods.

Less milk. A few of my patients, especially blacks, have complained of gassy indigestion for which all the usual measures gave little relief. This problem often stems from lack of an enzyme that breaks down curds formed in the stomach after ingestion of milk. About half of all blacks and 5 percent of whites have this condition and simply can't stay comfortable after drinking whole or skim milk. Most of these people can digest yogurt and cheese and some can digest ice cream. Butter generally causes no problem, since it contains milk fat without the offending protein. Since milk is an important source of calcium and other nutrients, you should test your response to the usually-tolerated milk products and stress them in your diet if they cause no distress. If all milk products bother you, take three calcium tablets (5 grain strength) a day to make up for the loss of that important bone-building nutrient. Calcium supplements are especially important during pregnancy and in growing children, but have some importance even when growing bones aren't adding extra calcium need.

How to fight a tendency toward indigestion. If you are subject to indigestion, you can take many effective steps right in your own home to prevent attacks from getting a start. Both morale-boosting and physical measures definitely help. You should either make mealtimes cheerful times or adjust your meals to fit your mood and circumstances, besides using physical correctives.

Check family and business problems at the dining room door. Mealtime should be a time of relaxed enjoyment. You certainly help digestion when you make mealtime more mentally relaxed and more socially enjoyable.

The vice-president of a large publishing house met me once for luncheon. We had a pleasant meal, during which we discussed everything from Broadway plays to dry fly fishing. Then we went to his office for a business chat. As I was leaving, he said:

"A few years ago, I would have done this differently. Instead of just passing the time of day at luncheon and killing another half an hour getting our business settled, I would have gotten down to business with the main course. We would have signed a contract before dessert. Then I would have come up here and wrestled with indigestion for a solid hour!"

I've seen so many patients who followed that same futile routine! They do it with business affairs: if there's nobody to dicker with, they work away with reports and timetables when they should be enjoying a calm lunch. They do it with family affairs: they bicker all the way through a meal instead of setting a cooperative mood with the quiet companionship of the dinner table and then discussing their differences later. They even do it with completely private worries, fretting themselves into indigestion when a pleasant mealtime interlude might help them try to find a fresh, productive approach. Wouldn't it be much better to do as my publisher friend now does? To use mealtime for pleasant personal exchange and relaxed enjoyment, then make a fresh attack upon your problems?

Build pleasant conversation. Properly guided conversation inevitably sets a good, digestion-aiding mood at mealtime. The trick is to lead your companions gently toward topics that interest or stimulate them. One of the best conversationalists I know blames his success on the morning newspaper, a red pencil, and a ten-minute wait between buses every day. He scans the paper quickly, learning just enough about each headline to know what it is about and whom it might interest.

"I don't know the answers," he says. "All I know is the right questions to ask or the right issues to raise."

That's all it takes to avoid dull silence, arguments or embarrassment during mealtimes. You can get your husband talking with a remark like, "Which do you think is the team to watch in pro football this year?" You can steer conversation away from a topic that might lead to hard feelings by referring to a new subject which interests the other person: the latest dress styles, or the effect of union racketeering on labor. Such a stock of fresh topics with which to draw out your companions takes only a few minutes a day to accumulate.

Make meals more alluring. You can help your stomach to make more of its precious digestive juice by making meals and mealtime more alluring. Actual measurements prove that the flow of gastric juices increases dramatically when you look at an appetizing meal. More gastric juices pour into your stomach when you *look* at attractively prepared food than when you actually *taste* it. This extra flow of gastric juice becomes more and more important as the years go by and stomach juices become scanty. Yet many people take less and less trouble with sprucing up their meals as they grow older.

Margaret Bradshaw was a good example. Her husband died when she was fifty. For the next four years, she was plagued by indigestion. Yet she was cheerful, had many friends and few worries.

Margaret Bradshaw was too busy making a new life to spend time fixing attractive meals for herself. When she took work as housekeeper-companion for an elderly relative, she conscientiously dressed up the meals she served for her employer and herself. Result: an almost instant end to indigestion.

Fit meals to your mood. When you are in the grip of any strong emotion, such as anger, fear or excitement, or if the circumstances in which you eat may lead to such feelings, you should not eat heavy or hard-to-digest foods. You can either delay meals or simplify and lighten them. One of my patients, for instance, had a violent temper and an acrimonious wife. For years, not only his household but also his abdomen were in perpetual uproar. But no longer. He has finally learned to skip meals when he is angry. He storms out of the house at least once a week, walks the streets until he calms down, then takes a bowl of cream-style soup every hour or two until his stomach stops churning. Without the miseries of indigestion, he is making real progress toward a more pleasant life.

Better teeth for good digestion. Frequent, severe attacks of indigestion often stem from poor teeth or inadequate chewing. Take Hilda Swanson's case, for example. At age sixty-three, Hilda was spending several hundred dollars a year at the drug store. Her life was a never-ending succession of poached eggs, milk toast, and misery. Heartburn and gas pains plagued her when she tried to eat solid foods, constipation tortured her when she didn't. Yet there was nothing wrong with Hilda's stomach or bowel. Half a dozen examinations and several X-rays had been entirely normal.

Poor Hilda! She spent so much on pills and potions that she had nothing left for her teeth. Her smile was a jagged horror. Only two pairs of teeth in her head met in any kind of bite. Her appearance finally drove her children into arranging for her dentist to fit her with plates. To everyone's surprise, her digestion improved overnight once she had effective teeth. Today, Hilda enjoys her food again. She hardly ever takes a pill, and thanks God that her children were worried about her jagged smile.

Food to fit your teeth. Suit your food choices to your teeth. If your teeth can't be fixed so that you can chew everything easily, you'll have to give in to them. Follow these simple rules:

1. Take hard-to-bite foods in a different form. Instead of eating a whole apple, have it cut up in salad or fruit cup.
2. Morsel food before eating it. If you get a tough piece of meat, cut a thin piece against the grain, then slice across it several times with the grain before gathering a bite with your fork.
3. Soften food in preparation. Get the butcher to tenderize meat and grind your hamburger twice. Have steaks thoroughly pounded before they are cooked. Be sure that vegetables are slightly overcooked to soften their fiber.

Take time to chew. Give yourself time to eat calmly, time to chew well, and time to enjoy your meals. I've seen many a case of indigestion cured by the simple advice to chew each bite at least ten times. The first week a patient follows this rule, he concentrates on counting. After that, he discovers flavor, leisurely enjoyment of food, new satisfaction at the table and misery-free digestion. He doesn't have to count any more. He chews automatically.

Low acidity indigestion. If you have stomach bloating, fullness, belching, and discomfort after meals, you may suffer from lack of stomach acid. Properly diluted hydrochloric acid just before and during meals often gives tremendous relief. Buy *dilute* hydrochloric acid, also called 0.1 N, at your drugstore, put ten drops in a glass of water and set it on the table with each meal. Sip the solution through a glass straw with its tip well inside your teeth on top of your tongue to avoid possible dental damage. Take a sip or two before beginning to eat, and repeat at intervals throughout the meal.

Caffeine-spurred indigestion. As few as three cups of coffee a day or equivalent amounts of tea or cola beverages can cause digestive disturbances over a period of time in sensitive people. Digestive effects are slow to appear and slow to leave: it takes three weeks of overindulgence to cause trouble, and almost as long to improve after you cut down on coffee-drinking. Patients who get well after a switch to decaffeinated coffee often had no indigestion until after age forty, even though they had been drinking lots of coffee since age twenty or so. They almost never complain of coffee nerves.

If there's any chance that caffeine might be troubling your digestion, switch to decaffeinated coffee for a month. You can continue to drink regular coffee in restaurants or in other people's homes so long as you keep it down to one or two cups a day. At the end of the first month, the harmful caffeine effects should be about gone. See whether the next week or two are brightened by better digestion. If they are, keep dodging excess caffeine for life.

Worms. When I first started in practice, I remember puzzling over one of the Olson brood. Young Sam had stomach aches and side aches two or three times a week. He didn't eat heartily the way a twelve-year-old should. But his blood count and x-rays were perfectly all right, and I couldn't seem to find a cure.

One day the boy's grandmother was confined to bed, so I went out to see her. The house was spic and span, without a speck of dirt, and Grandma was propped between snowy sheets. I checked her out and prescribed for her. As I got ready to leave, her daughter asked me to take a look at Sam, who was having "another of his attacks." I looked the boy over and suggested another crop of x-rays.

"X-rays?" Grandmother snorted from her sickbed. "Why in my day we'd have cured that boy six months ago. Give him a good slug of worm medicine and that would be the end of it."

You know what? She was one hundred per cent right! Knowing how scrubbed and spic and span the Olson house was, it never occurred to me that young Sam might have worms. But I know better now, and the first thing I do when a youngster complains of stomach pains or loss of appetite is check a bit of stool under the microscope to see if it contains worm eggs. It happens in the best of families, and without anyone making any breach in cleanliness or proper care!

Prescription measures work so much better than home remedies on the various types of worms that I'm not going to advise how you can treat them. But doctors are squeamish about checking for this condition, especially when they know you run a clean household and might be offended by the suggestion. You often have to take the initiative in getting the proper studies done. Particularly if your youngster has suggestive complaints or if you live in a warm, moist climate, catch a bit of stool and take it in when any of your youngsters sees a doctor. You'll be surprized at how often stubborn, smoldering difficulties stem from easily cured infestation with worms.

HOME CARE FOR ULCERS AND GASTRITIS

If you get heartburn or boring pain in the pit of your stomach at least once a day an hour or two after meals, you probably have either gastritis or an ulcer. Any digestive complaints which last more than three weeks deserve a medical checkup, of course. However, prompt home care may get the problem under control before expensive X-rays and doctor visits become worthwhile. Exactly the same home care often cures either gastritis or beginning ulcer, so you can use these remedies whenever you have suggestive complaints:

Simplified ulcer-healing diet. You can usually bring an ulcer or attack of gastritis under control promptly by taking six small meals of very bland foods a day. Eat cooked cereal, soft boiled or poached eggs, toast, butter, strained cream soups, custards, puddings, or plain cookies. You can eat ice cream, too, if you let it melt in your mouth before you swallow it.

Acid-absorbing milk. While you are healing your ulcer or gastritis, you need something to neutralize stomach acids as quickly as they form. Milk is the best answer. Half a glass of whole milk or of half-milk-half-cream every hour except at mealtime does the trick. For a change-off and at bedtime, try yogurt. This has the same acid-neutralizing and nutritional qualities as milk and a variety of flavors. The more solid consistency helps to keep it in your stomach a little longer, which is especially helpful for neutralizing night acids.

Antacids. If the six-feeding diet and the milk portions between do not keep you entirely comfortable, try aluminum hydroxide tablets between milk feedings. These tablets are available without prescription under various brand names such as "Gelusil" and "Amphogel." Chew well and take them with water. As your condition improves, you still need something to neutralize stomach acids every 90 minutes during the day for several weeks. Aluminum hydroxide often proves much more convenient than milk. Try it at first alternating with milk, then as your acid-fighting mainstay.

Milk of magnesia. With little solid food and lots of constipating milk and medicine, most gastritis victims find that their bowels get rather tight. Since milk of magnesia acts both as an antacid and as a mild laxative, you can usually keep your bowels going by replacing one or two doses of aluminum hydroxide with milk of magnesia each day. Don't strive for daily movements, though. As long as the material is easily passed and is formed in normal sausage shapes, even two movements a week are sufficient.

Convalescent diet. After you have freed yourself of digestive discomfort for a week, you can usually go back to a three meal program. You should probably stay off of seasonings, spices, and alcohol for good. Let hot foods cool somewhat before eating them and let cold foods warm in your mouth before you swallow. Choose stewed or roasted meat over broiled whenever possible, and avoid fried foods altogether. Try to get your vegetables cooked a bit longer than usual so that they will be soft, and chew them thoroughly. Keep taking at least one glassful of milk between meals and in the evening for several months or years.

How to keep an ulcer from coming back. If you have a tendency toward ulcer or gastritis, you can usually take effective measures to keep further attacks from plaguing you.

Precautions under stress. When you know that you are under extra emotional stress or when you get into an upsetting situation, you can often ward off an ulcer attack by anticipating it. In mildly distressing situations, simply eating half a cup of yogurt at bedtime each night may do the trick. Night acids are the first to increase when an ulcer threatens, and yogurt sticks in the stomach long enough to neutralize at least the worst of these. In times of greater stress, go on your full six meal program with milk or antacid every hour for two or three days. That's easier than letting the ulcer get a fresh start.

Build an ulcer-dodging way of life. Even the worst ulcers can be prevented by a happy choice of attitude. That's what an Iowa internist proved a few years ago when he got tired of treating the same patients over and over again for ulcers. He picked the very worst cases, people who had suffered at least three recent bouts with ulcer. Then he asked each of them something like this:

"Want to spend one night a month trying to keep from getting another attack? No pills, no shots, no treatments: just come in for a quiet chat with some other people who have the same sort of problems. Together, maybe you can work out a better way to reduce or meet the stresses of life.''

Over thirty patients took him up on it. They met after normal office hours and talked about effectual, contented living. Seven years later, my friend counted up the score. Without the conferences, these patients should have suffered at least forty ulcer bouts, many of them severe. With the conferences, only four mild attacks had developed.

You can promote ulcer-dodging, digestion-improving attitudes in yourself. Only extreme cases, like the ulcer-ridden unfortunates my Iowa friend assembled, need expert help in working out a new viewpoint. You can probably decide for yourself whether your attitudes need any changes, and if so act accordingly.

Decide how much to depend on others emotionally and how much to let them depend on you. The main key to freedom from digestion-wrecking stress is just the right balance between self-reliance on the one hand, and genuine concern for others and need for their loving support on the other. You need to feel that others depend on you. You also need to depend on *them*—to yearn for and receive evidence of their concern.

You can easily develop such two-way support and need without losing control of your own destiny or confidence in your own powers. The secret is compassion: emotional sharing of each other's trials. Advice and even actual aid are sometimes threats: they can hamper self-reliance and destroy self-confidence. Compassion is no threat. You can feel for others and let them know that you are behind them without taking over their decisions or putting them in your debt. You can share and discuss feelings which upset you without asking advice or aid.

How Bill Harper built himself a web of ulcer-healing emotional bonds. Bill Harper wore all the trappings of success when he first visited my office: a tailored suit, a diamond ring, and the miserable, drawn expression of perennial ulcer suffering.

"I've always been a battler," he told me toward the end of his visit. "I've fought for business, fought for social position, fought for community standing. Why should that give me an ulcer, though? I usually win!"

"Fighting for things doesn't cause ulcers," I told him. "It's the insecurity that makes you *have* to fight. What makes you a battler? Why can't you enjoy the fruits of each success instead of moving on?"

"I can't answer that. I'm just that kind of a guy."

"Don't you think some of your drive comes from dissatisfaction? How about your family life, for instance?"

"I'm proud of my family—I'd do anything for them, and they'd do anything for me."

"Is that enough?"

Bill Harper looked at me thoughtfully. "I'll think about that," he said, and left.

The next time we talked about family life was nearly a year afterward.

"My wife made me very happy today," Bill said.

"How?" I asked.

"She told me what has been troubling her recently. She's worried sick about our girl going steady already at age seventeen."

He smiled ruefully, then went on:

"A year ago she wouldn't have come to me. And if she had, I wouldn't have known what to do, except send them both on a trip to Bermuda or something. We've come a long way since then: she told me because she knew I'd be concerned, and I guess we both felt better afterward."

Bill Harper hasn't had any more trouble with his ulcer. He's found new, lasting satisfaction in his home, with truly deep emotional attachments to replace the selfish, pragmatic pride of yesteryear. The same change improves his friendships and even his business contacts. Without in any way decreasing his success, he's put his life on a sounder emotional footing, and enjoyed both psychological and physical benefits.

Learn to say "no." Next to proper balance of self-reliance and close, mutual concern, the most important key to freedom from digestion-wrecking stress is ability to say "no." It's altogether too easy to drift into a harried, over-burdened ineffectiveness by saying "yes" to whatever anyone asks you to do.

A distinguished community leader and old family friend made this point for me in an unexpected way. When I was in my twenties, he asked me to take on a responsibility I didn't want. I hated to refuse such an old and respected friend, so I hedged. After several miserable days of stalling, I finally said "no."

"Thank Heaven!" my friend replied. "You've finally arrived."

"What do you mean?" I asked.

"You've taken your place as a man. Until the day you first say 'no' to someone or something you like, you're just a piece of human jetsam, floating with the tides of man's demands. Now you're setting your own course. Congratulations!"

That moment comes back to me whenever I see an overburdened sufferer from abdominal distress. To get him well more quickly, I usually tell him to stop all of his activities and responsibilities except one or two. Then as he starts to pick up the threads again, I say:

"Pick and choose. Of course you want to help everybody who asks, but you can't. So figure all the responsibilities you have—family, business, household, and community—before you take on a new job or join another group. Can you add this without taking away from something else? If not, what do you want to drop to make room for it?

"Ask yourself these questions, and you'll find yourself saying 'no' to many offers. But don't feel badly about it. You're giving yourself more thoroughly, as well as enjoying yourself much more, if you stick to the jobs which really fit you as a person, and fit your stores of energy and time."

Most harried, dyspeptic people find this advice worthwhile. Does it suit your situation?

Evade or rid yourself of resentment. You can frequently ease some digestion-wrecking stress by evading or releasing resentment. Several years ago, Drs. Wolf and Wolfe studied digestion in a patient who had an opening directly into his stomach. The man was hired as a janitor at the hospital, partly so that he would be available for the doctors' experiments. He wasn't a very good janitor: he was often called on the carpet. But that seemed to make very little difference to his stomach.

Then one day, it did make a difference. The inside of his stomach was beet-red in places, blotchy, sensitive and raw.

"What's happened to you, Tom?" the doctors asked.

"Just a bawling out," the patient said. But further questioning revealed one special point: this bawling out was for something not his fault. This bawling out he deeply resented, knowing it was undeserved, while he had taken others as a matter of course.

Is your stomach ever upset, sensitive, and uncomfortable? If so, seek back for sources of resentment. You'll find that you will want to dodge some similar stresses in the future as simply not worth the upsetting effect they have on you. Other resentments fade when you talk them over with your family or friends. Still others rankle until you develop some safety-valve activity—a hobby or sports interest that lets you cut or chop, hit a ball, or shoot a pheasant. Emotion ceases to cause ulcers when it has an easy outlet, even though that outlet is through conversation or assault on wood or leather. For complete details, see pages 235–236.

BILIOUS INDIGESTION, AND GALL BLADDER DISEASE AND STONE

Bilious indigestion responds very well to simple home measures, as long as you do not have true gall-bladder colic. Colic shows up as cramp-like pain below the edge of your right ribs. The cramps come about every two minutes and last ten seconds or so (although it seems much longer). They may run through to your back, right under your shoulder blade. Nausea or vomiting often adds its miseries to the colicky pain. Since gallstones frequently underlie attacks of colic, prompt prescription measures are definitely worthwhile once cramps occur. Otherwise, home treatment may bring your problem promptly under control.

Bilious indigestion. When you get gas cramps, bloating, and belching after eating fried food or pork, your difficulty may be bilious indigestion. Many patients get considerable relief from home measures.

Enemas and suppositories. A carminative enema (one quart of water at 115 degrees with two teaspoonfuls of spirits of peppermint), followed by a Wyanoid suppository gives prompt relief from most bilious attacks (For further details see p. 68.) Prescription type spasm soothers may give benefit, too.

Low fat diet. A low fat diet helps ward off further attacks of bilious indigestion. Fried foods, pork, rich pastries, and oil-containing dressings must go. Replace cream with half and half, avoid whipping cream and keep butter down to one or two pats a day. Eat plenty of lean broiled or boiled meat, vegetables, and fruit.

Bile salts. Some patients find that they get considerable relief from bile salts (Bilron, Anabile, or any of several other brands). One tablet with each meal usually helps to keep the bowels active and prevents some bloating and gas pain. These tablets cause no heartburn or bitter belching if you take them during the meal rather than on an empty stomach and swallow them whole. *But* remember that so-called liver pills are *not* adequate sources of bile salts, and are not recommended.

Laxative salts. You get better bile flow as well as relief from constipation with a dose of Phospho-soda or Epsom salts. Although these agents should not usually be used for ordinary constipation (see Chapter Four), they work very effectively for the constipation that accompanies biliousness. In fact, the effect on bile flow probably makes a dose worthwhile whenever you miss your movement for 48 hours, if bilious indigestion is continually with you.

Serious gall bladder trouble. If you get proper medical care at the first sign of gall bladder colic, you may actually escape the need for surgery. As long as gallstones are very small or the gall bladder is only inflamed instead of packed with stones, your doctor may be able to prescribe diet and medicines that will help.

How to make a gall bladder operation easier to bear. If other methods fail or if your case is not suited to them, an operation almost always cures gall bladder trouble. You can make this operation much safer and easier to bear in three ways:

  1. Get medical treatment from the start. Some people suffer through one attack of gallstone colic after another without a doctor's help because they are

afraid that as soon as they call a doctor, he will operate. A doctor's help during and after early attacks may ward off the need for surgery. If it doesn't do that, it will keep you in good condition to undergo operation with less risks and difficulties.

2. Lose any excess weight. As soon as you have any suspicion that your gall bladder may be causing trouble, use the suggestions in Chapter 18 to help you lose excess weight. If you are overweight, the risks and miseries of surgery can be cut in half simply by getting to normal weight beforehand.

3. Go ahead with the operation before complications arise. Gallstones can work into the main bile passages, causing jaundice and other severe problems. I've never seen a patient who had severe complications without several preceding gallstone colics. If you heed your body's painful warnings and your doctor's sound advice, you can avoid these extra miseries, risks and disabilities.

How Mrs. Simpson made her operation easier to bear. Olive Simpson was crying when I first saw her.

"It's not the pain," she said as she dabbed at her eyes with the corner of her handkerchief. "I'm just scared. My sister had her gall bladder out, and she had such an awful time!"

Olive had gall bladder colic which was due to large-sized stones. She needed an operation to get a cure, but her first attack settled down promptly. She had plenty of time to lose weight and get ready for surgery. When Olive went to the hospital four months later, she had lost forty pounds. She was as strong and healthy as she had ever been (her sister had waited until she was weak with jaundice).

"No operation is a picnic," Olive told me afterwards. "But when I think of what my sister went through, I'm mighty grateful for the easy time I had. There was just one day when I needed shots to ease my pain after surgery, and I got back on my feet in a tenth of the time it took her."

6

How to Heal Rectal and Bladder Complaints with Home Measures

There's no misery quite like the misery you get from rectal and bladder troubles, as every sufferer knows. Elimination complaints drag on and on until you think they'll never quit. Most of the commonest ones will yield to simple home measures, though. You can win considerable ease for yourself if you are plagued by hemorrhoids, rectal itching, rectal-opening splits, rectal aftermaths of childbearing or certain bladder ailments.

HOW TO SOOTHE HEMORRHOIDS AT HOME

Home measures can help you to soothe hemorrhoids to slow their formation or growth, and to make any doctoring they require more comfortable and less expensive. You need surgery for lasting, total cure once hemorrhoids have fully developed, but you can often keep them from reaching that point.

How to soothe clotted hemorrhoids. You can control most discomfort from hemorrhoids with simple home measures. When a hemorrhoid becomes painful, the bulged-out vein inside it usually has become stopped up with a blood clot. This results in swelling, which stretches the sensitive bowel lining or skin. When hemorrhoids hurt, you should try to help your body soak up the clot inside them and try to shrink or soothe the swollen tissue. You can definitely help your body soak up blood clots faster with hot water applied to the painful parts.

Hot towels. Fold an ordinary bath towel until it is six or eight layers thick. Wet it in hot water (about 112 degrees F), and wring it partly dry. Lie face down and place the towel between the buttocks so that it rests against the rectal area. Cover with a dry towel or piece of plastic film to cut down heat loss by evaporation, and dip again as soon as cooling begins. Continue for 20 minutes by the clock.

Hot sitz baths. A frequently more convenient and equally effective method of treating sore hemorrhoids spread through the western world from old-time Germany, where it was known as the "sitzenbad" or sitting bath. Somebody goofed in the course of translation, and the mythical Dr. Sitz has been getting credit for the invention ever since. The technique is simply to sit in about four inches of hot water for exactly 20 minutes. Wrap a towel around your shoulders so that you will not get chilled. Add hot water as required to keep the temperature at 112 degrees. If you do not have an accurate candy or darkroom thermometer, test the water with your hand frequently while heating it up: after your less sensitive parts become accustomed to heat, they sometimes give you no warning even when you add enough hot water to cause a burn. Let a little water out if the depth gets much above four inches: you want to draw more circulation to the sore rectal area, not to the whole surface of your skin.

Irritated hemorrhoids. If hemorrhoids are raw or itchy and not truly painful, try *zinc oxide ointment*. You can get this at your drugstore without prescription. Scoop up a thick glob with an enema tip or with the end of a soft rubber catheter. Insert the instrument gently just into the rectum and withdraw. Apply further ointment to the surface hemorrhoids. A covering film of cotton helps to keep ointment off your clothing.

Suppositories. Wyanoid or Anusol suppositories sometimes help when zinc oxide fails. Unwrap and insert suppositories blunt end first, immediately after each bowel movement.

Increasing or newly formed hemorrhoids. You can often make hemorrhoids subside or substantially slow their growth. The effective home measures you can apply for this purpose also improve your rectal comfort. Try this two-pronged attack:

1. Keep veins at the rectal opening from becoming over-engorged. You can often prevent hemorrhoids altogether or markedly slow their growth if you can keep the veins at the rectal opening from becoming over-engorged. Some of the web of veins in this area lead back to the heart through vessels inside the abdomen which branch many times within your liver. Others take a direct route to the heart without going through the abdominal cavity. When you increase the pressure on the veins inside your abdomen by straining at stool, lifting, stooping or coughing, you squeeze blood back from the veins inside the abdomen through the veins near the rectal opening into the free-flowing direct vein passage. Heavy flow of blood under high pressure in the small rectal veins is like heavy truck traffic on a dirt detour; it overloads and damages delicate vein walls.

You can prevent this whole chain of hemorrhoid-forming events by keeping down the pressure within your abdominal cavity. Three approaches are completely practical within your own home:

a. Learn to lift, stoop, and squat without squeezing or grunting. Let open, easy breathing serve as a constant safety valve against built-up abdominal pressures. At first, you will have to train yourself to keep breathing during muscular exertion: deliberately breathe in through your nose and out through your mouth as you lift, squat, stoop, or strain. Later, when this has become a habit, you will find that it not only helps preserve your rectal comfort but also increases your capacity for heavy work.

b. Avoid undue straining at stool. If a movement is very difficult, take a slow-action oil enema (see page 65) instead of proceeding. Follow the constipation control program outlined in Chapter Four for strain-free elimination.

c. Keep effective cough medicine on hand. Even if you could bear up under cough miseries, you can spare your rectum by controlling them.

2. Keep hard passages from aggravating hemorrhoids. When hemorrhoidal veins bulge out, they push the delicate bowel lining or skin into the bowel passage. Bruising and pulling further stretch and irritate the bulged-out tissue. The discomfort of movements leads to spasm, which allows the next movement to get extra hard. Difficult movements lead to pain, spasm, and still more pain: a vicious circle of misery and increasing harm.

If you suffer even slightly from hemorrhoids, you should take steps to keep this vicious circle from making them worse. The constipation cure from Chapter Four is very much worthwhile, but hemorrhoid sufferers should take these extra steps:

1. Get a soft rubber catheter, size 24 or 28, from your drugstore or surgical supply house. Use it in place of the usual hard rubber tip whenever you need an enema. Use lubricating jelly instead of petroleum jelly on the catheter, since petroleum jelly rots rubber. Insert only an inch or two for ordinary enemas, up to six or eight inches for oil.

2. Instill one ounce of olive or mineral oil into the rectum at bedtime whenever no bowel movement has occurred for two or more days. An all rubber ear syringe, which you can get at any drugstore for about a dollar, makes this procedure very easy and comfortable.

3. Take plain Metamucil, Surfak or a similar moist-bulk providing agent regularly in doses large enough to produce at least one movement every two days, if natural rhythm regulation makes for less frequent stools.

Protruding hemorrhoids. If a too-firm bowel movement pulls hemorrhoids from inside the rectal opening, you should slide them back in place promptly. Smooth pressure through several layers of toilet paper may do the trick. Lubricate the hemorrhoids with olive or mineral oil on a cotton ball if necessary. When discomfort is considerable, the muscle which cuts off the flow of bowel discharges has become tight around the hemorrhoids. Soothe the area with several minutes of hot applications for easier replacement of the protruding piles. Hot, wet towels or sitting in four inches of hot water works quite well.

When your doctor's help is worthwhile for hemorrhoids. If you have hemorrhoids, you usually need a doctor's help to prove that you have no serious underlying condition. You often need his help to achieve a complete and lasting cure.

Anything which causes enlargement or change in an abdominal organ, from preganancy or ovarian cyst to rectal cancer or liver disease, can cause detouring of blood through the veins at the rectal opening and make hemorrhoids form. If hemorrhoids bleed in such a way that blood mixes in through the stool instead of merely showing on the paper, or if there are other signs of internal disorder such as change in bowel habit, weight loss, or pencil-shaped, small stools, you have an excellent chance of stopping a serious disorder, before it gets a foothold, by seeing your doctor promptly. You can usually put off examination for hemorrhoids that only bleed on the paper until your next visit to a doctor for some other complaint. Ask for a complete rectal examination at that time: your doctor can usually tell without putting you to any extra expense or inconvenience whether any underlying problem is present.

Injection treatments or operation usually gives complete and permanent cure for hemorrhoids. If all your hemorrhoids originate inside the rectal opening, when you see your doctor you can usually avoid operation altogether. At this stage, internal hemorrhoids yield to painless injection treatments or to rubber band ligature done in your doctor's office instead of in the hospital. If your condition does call for an operation, though, don't let old wives' tales frighten you: today's methods of pain relief and gentleness will positively keep you from suffering severe discomfort.

Sore hemorrhoids as large as or larger than the tip of your thumb or hemorrhoids which fail to subside with heat and ointment deserve the prompt relief your doctor can give.

HOW TO RELIEVE RECTAL ITCHING

The secret of curing ordinary rectal itching, whether you have hemorrhoids or not, is to soothe the irritation caused by material which seeps out from the bowel. After each bowel movement, take these four steps:

1. Cleanse the rectal area with soap and warm water on a soft washcloth. Follow with several spongings of plain water to rinse away the soap. This

procedure is much less irritating than rubbing raw, scratch-scored skin with any kind of paper, even facial tissue.

2. Sponge off entire area with rubbing alcohol. This kills germs and helps dry the macerated skin.

3. Powder the area with talc or cornstarch. A drying powder helps the skin to resist itch-producing fluids which seep out of the rectum.

4. Take a wisp of cotton about half as big as a cigarette, powder it with talc or cornstarch, smooth it over the tip of your index finger and insert it about half an inch into the rectal opening just far enough so that it will stay in place. This acts as a wick to prevent seepage. If large hemorrhoids are present, you may need to make the piece of cotton somewhat larger and put it a bit farther into the opening to keep it in place.

How to cure rectal dermatitis at home. If rectal itching is severe and application of rubbing alcohol burns or stings badly, your case has probably reached the stage of rectal dermatitis. Apply cloths wet with Burow's solution three or four times a day for ten minutes. You can get either tablets or concentrate with which to make Burow's solution from your druggist without a prescription. Use one tablet or one tablespoonful of concentrate to a pint of lukewarm water. After two to four days of applying Burow's you can usually switch to the alcohol-talc-wick method used for ordinary itching.

Malt soup extract. A few victims of rectal itching or dermatitis find that they can rid themselves of this misery altogether with malt soup extract. You will find this material at the infant feeding section of your drugstore instead of in with the medicines. Take one tablespoonful either mixed with cereal or stirred in water with each of your three meals.

When your doctor can help with rectal itching. Your doctor can give worthwhile aid for rectal itching under several different circumstances:

1. Rectal itching after bedtime often means pinworms, especially in households with preschool and early-grade youngsters. About one-third of children in this age group have pinworms. Adults in their families often become involved. Fortunately, piperazine (antepar) cures most cases permanently without the mess and bother of enemas and other measures which old-fashioned treatment usually required.

2. Persistent cases get relief with hydrocortisone ointment recently released by the F.D.A. for nonprescription use.

3. Rectal itching associated with pain, discomfort, or bulging usually is due to some underlying condition such as a split at the bowel opening or hemorrhoids. The underlying disorder may need medical treatment before you get relief.

PINWORMS

I'll stack Minnesota households against any in the world for cleanliness. Yet I've seen as many as forty percent of the youngsters in a Minnesota kindergarten prove to have pinworms. In fact, I've gotten to the point where any preschool youngster in my office who squirms and pulls at clothing in his body creases gets a test for this condition immediately. Squirming and restlessness are easier to spot than itching—youngsters often don't zero in on discomforts precisely and may not really "scratch where it itches"—but scratching around the seat or vaginal irritation may also point to pinworm problems.

Home check for pinworms. When your youngsters are in their soundest sleep, usually between eleven and twelve at night, mother pinworm crawls out of the rectum and lays her eggs. This is the source of all that later itching, squirming and discomfort—and you can catch her at her work if you just look. You'll find that you can expose the rectal area and look very thoroughly without even rousing your sleeping preschooler (or early-elementary-schooler). If present, the worms look like little bits of white thread about half an inch in length. They will often be in folds and creases, so you will need to spread the skin slightly in different directions in order to spot them. Use a bright flashlight for further aid.

Doctor tests for pinworms. Your doctor can't tell whether or not pinworms are present by examining a specimen of stool. The easiest way with youngsters is to stick some Scotch tape over the rectal area, peel it off, and examine it under the microscope. When growth of hair makes this test impractical, gentle skin scrapings work best.

Treatment. Pinworms build up by vicious-circle action. Eggs laid on the skin cause itching, scratching gets eggs on the hands and from there they get back into the mouth either on food or through thumb-sucking, etc. You can clear up the problem over a long period of time by keeping the child's fingernails trimmed down close and keeping him or her clothed (especially at night) in a way which makes it impossible to scratch.

For quick results, though, there are no home measures to match prescription ones. The usual prescription remedy (piperazine) is both highly effective and free of unpleasant side effects. One problem: pinworm eggs in their dry form float all over the house and usually affect everyone in it to some degree. If you go the quick, medicinal route, best treat everyone in the family at once (including the adults) to keep the untreated ones from reinfecting the rest.

RECTAL SPLITS AND FISSURES

You can almost always cure the commonest painful condition at the rectal opening for yourself in your own home and avoid the need for rectal surgery if you take action promptly. A split in the surface layer of the rectal opening causes considerable discomfort. Your first warning is often a tearing sensation followed by burning pain, which occurs during the passage of a hard stool. In other cases, pain may increase gradually, usually beginning at the conclusion of a movement and lasting 30 seconds to five minutes. After the onset of the rectal split, movements cause some burning discomfort during the passage of stool and red-hot-poker pain immediately thereafter. Since any form of rectal pain usually tightens the bowel, constipation aggravates the problem.

Severe discomfort after bowel movements almost always means a rectal split. Take these steps promptly for surgery-saving home cure:

1. Assure soft, easily passed movements while the rectal split heals. Take a tablespoonful of *Metamucil* twice daily, mixing each with one glass of water and following with another. Get a two-ounce all-rubber ear syringe. Fill it with *olive or mineral* oil. At bedtime, insert the soft rubber tip just inside the rectum. Slowly squeeze the oil into the bowel cavity. Withdraw the syringe, and put a sanitary pad (as Kotex) or pad of cotton in place to catch any oil which seeps out during the night. Use full-sized, six-ounce slow action oil enemas (see page 65) at night if movements do not occur daily, and follow with a *salt and soda enema* given through a soft rubber catheter rather than an ordinary enema tip if no movement has occurred by 10 o'clock the next morning (see page 68).

2. Soothe the split at the rectal opening. Put a glob of *zinc oxide ointment* on the tip of the ear syringe when you take your nightly stool-softening treatment. Apply zinc oxide ointment in a similar way twice during the day. If the split is very sore, use Surfacaine ointment or Nupercainal for a few days instead of zinc oxide.

3. Relieve spasm in the muscle which cuts off the flow of bowel contents. Use soothing heat three times a day by applying *hot wet towels* or taking sitz baths. If pain or muscle spasm persists, use astringent or antispasmodic (Anusol or Wyanoid) suppositories every 12 hours. Unwrap and insert each suppository blunt end first.

This home program for healing rectal splits will almost always do the trick in four weeks. If a rectal split already has a head start or fails to respond to home measures, your doctor can heal it for you with surgery. The operation required is not an unusually painful one. It can sometimes be done without hospitalization, and never requires more than a day or two of hospital care.

HOME MEASURES A WOMAN CAN USE FOR CYSTOCOEL AND RECTOCOEL

You can often prevent or control by prompt action the two commonest special female problems of elimination which otherwise lead to years of nagging discomfort, and often to ultimate surgery. These conditions arise through bulging of the rectum or the bladder into the female organ. Rectocoel or cystocoel usually plagues women whose tissues have been stretched in childbirth, although childless women are not immune. Both conditions are usually present in severe cases.

How to control rectocoel or cystocoel. Proper elimination keeps down strain on the thin walls of tissue which separate the rectum and bladder from the female opening. Even if you already suffer from slipping and sliding sensations or slight bulging, these steps may keep rectocoel and cystocoel under control:

1. Prevent bulge-forming abdominal pressures by controlling constipation and severe cough. Follow the program for constipation outlined in Chapter Four. Get prescription-strength (½ grain of codeine per dose) cough syrup from your doctor when you get a severe cold.

2. Heed nature's calls. An over-full bladder presses down and stretches the wall between it and the vagina. A bowel movement which has become difficult through unwarranted delay places strain on the tissues which divide the rectum from the female canal. You can avoid both unnecessary strains by heeding nature's calls promptly.

3. Empty your bowels in a posture which directs the advancing stool directly out the rectum opening or to the rear of it. When you sit upright with your feet flat on the floor, the advancing stool drives into the wall between rectum and vagina. This flimsy wall must turn it toward the proper opening. The least tendency to be swaybacked increases this problem tremendously: arch the lower portion of your back forward, and you will see how hollow-backed posture directs material from the abdomen toward the front of the elimination tube. You can correct these problems in three easy ways: You can roll your pelvis forward as you sit, as if you were trying to look at the female opening during the movement. You can increase the bend of your knees and the fold of your hips by putting your feet on a high footstool and leaning well forward or by clasping your arms around your knees during actions. Or you can learn to squat on the toilet rim with the

seat up, which directs the advancing stool properly in almost every single case.

One of my patients, for instance, complained that she could not expel a bowel movement except by pressing her fingers against the back of her vagina. When she assumed her usual sway-backed sitting posture, the reason was all too clear: material moving down her rectum had to turn nearly a right angle on its way to the outer opening. The flimsy recto-vaginal wall was not strong enough to deflect firm movements, so a tremendous forward bulge had formed. Surgery was the only answer by that time, but the whole chain of events could have been prevented or ameliorated if she had learned to empty her bowels in a flexed posture some years before.

4. Strengthen separations between various openings with pelvic exercises. Any woman who has had a child should build the strength of her pelvic muscles. You can do pelvic exercises either sitting up or lying down, in the privacy of your own home or while you are riding on the bus to work: wherever you have a few moments undisturbed. First, try to squeeze the female opening together with its own musculature, as if you were picking up marbles with it. Hold the muscles contracted for three to five seconds, then relax. Next, try to lift the bowel opening straight up into the pelvis. Hold it for three to five seconds, then relax. Continue alternating these two kinds of contraction of pelvic musculature for about two minutes. Follow this routine three times a day for three to four weeks to build pelvic muscle strength, then once a day to maintain it. (This same exercise greatly increases your capacity to satisfy your husband sexually. Not only does it make for snugger union, but it teaches voluntary control. After you get the muscles built up, try pumping them rapidly in this same order during sexual relations, or squeezing and relaxing the vagina at the sex climax. Your husband will love you for it!)

5. Drink plenty of extra water. Besides bulging discomforts, cystocoel frequently causes bladder irritation. This causes you to have to urinate frequently, often with little advance notice or urge. Burning discomfort on urination may also plague you. You can usually stave off this kind of trouble by keeping the urinary passages flushed out with copious urinary flow. About two extra quarts a day of water, fruit juice or non-cola containing beverages usually do the trick.

When your doctor can give worthwhile help with rectocoel and cystocoel. Your doctor can usually arrange relief for you if you suffer from rectocoel or cystocoel. Sometimes a supporting internal brace helps. In more severe cases, operation gives fairly thorough relief. Surgery is quite safe and does not keep you inactive for very long.

HOME CARE FOR CYSTITIS

The shortness and breadth of the tube from the bladder to the exterior makes women particularly subject to cystitis, although some men suffer from it, too. Attacks usually start with burning and stinging on urination. The urge to void becomes frequent, sometimes every five minutes. Victims often complain that they will feel an unrequited urge after voiding. Urine usually looks cloudy or smoky, and sometimes appears bloody, too. This condition may cause one or two degrees of fever.

Home care for early and mild cystitis. The germs which start a bladder infection often die out if you change the chemical character of your urine through simple home measures. This is particularly true at the very beginning of infection, when very few germs have had a chance to burrow into the bladder wall and virtually all are still bathed in urine. Take these two steps at the very first sign of burning, frequent urination, or a sense of being unable to empty the bladder:

1. Drink copious amounts of water, ginger ale, orange juice, or lemonade. Try to down at least three or four extra quarts of fluid each day. You'll find you can drink more by taking a small juice glass every 10 or 15 minutes than by trying to choke down a whole glassful every hour. Moderately chilled drinks usually pass through the stomach more quickly than ice cold ones, too.

2. Take two teaspoonfuls of baking soda in a little water every two hours during waking hours for two or three days, provided you have no heart or kidney trouble. Do not take this step if your doctor has told you to avoid excess salt: the sodium ion, which is what he wants you to avoid, is contained in baking soda as well as table salt.

Spasm-soothing suppositories. Wyanoids suppositories, Donnatal, Doan's Pills or medically prescribed spasm soothers often give considerable relief from cystitis. They do not speed your cure particularly, but they relieve discomfort and allow a longer interval between voidings.

How to ward off toilet paper cystitis. Germs often get a big head start in moving from the intestinal opening to the bladder by faulty cleansing technique. You can carry a positive horde of cystitis-causing germs forward to the urinary outlet with one forward stroke of the toilet paper. This very common source of bladder infection is easy to dodge: simply avoid reaching between your legs to cleanse your rectal opening, keeping your cleaning motions to the rectal area itself instead of including the genital zone, and use each tissue for only one front-to-back stroke.

Honeymoon cystitis. Another common aid to cystitis germs on their passage up the urinary tract is sexual activity. Intercourse in positions where the man's angle of entrance directs the penis toward the front of the vagina catches the urinary tube against the inside of the pelvic bones and milks germs along it. Although these positions give great satisfaction at times, they predispose toward cystitis during periods of very frequent intercourse, such as a honeymoon or reunion after a long absence.

Sex position during highly active periods. Whenever you expect to have relations more than three times a week, you should avoid sex postures in which the man's angle of entrance brings the penis snugly against the front wall of the vagina. The only two common postures in which this occurs are the folded hip postures, in which the woman folds her hips after entry and either hooks her heels on her husband's shoulders or pulls her knees up close to her armpits. The standard position and woman's-legs-down-straight position put absolutely no strain on the bladder, and can be used freely during frequent-sex periods.

Drink plenty of water. Adequate flow of urine helps to flush away any germs that get close to your bladder. If you heed your body's thirst signals, this need is ordinarily met. I have seen several women who developed bladder infections after cutting down on liquids at and after supper in order to avoid getting up at night to urinate. Certainly, such limitation is most unwise during lively-sex weeks.

When your doctor can give worthwhile help with cystitis. Thanks to today's large assortment of powerful germ-killing medicines, your doctor can almost always cure cystitis in a matter of hours. You don't need to suffer along for days if home measures fail to help you.

Even if home measures are effective against cystitis, your doctor's help is worthwhile in two instances:

When you have passed blood in your urine, special examinations are necessary. Many of the urinary disorders whose first warning is bloody urine yield much more readily to prompt than to delayed treatment. Since these conditions may mimic bladder infection quite closely, anyone who passes blood should have a complete examination of the bladder and kidneys.

A man who has two attacks or a woman who has three attacks of cystitis should have special examinations to search for a smoldering source of infection or an abnormality which makes him especially liable to urinary disease. This examination should at least include special kidney X-rays, and usually also an examination of the inside of the bladder. Doctors can identify and cure almost all of the conditions that lead to repeated urinary infections at this stage, whereas they might not be able to do so later.

Bedwetting. "I don't know what we're going to do with George,"

Clarice said, shooing her ten-year-old toward my examining table. "He's scheduled to go to church camp next month, and he's still wetting the bed."

Attempting to shame a youngster out of bedwetting often backs the whole family into a corner. My heart went out to young George, who obviously wished he could find a crack to crawl into. But at this point he needed something more than sympathy.

"Does he have to strain for a long time to get the stream started when he urinates?" I asked. "Some youngsters have a flap of tissue or a constriction in the tube out from the bladder and have a hard time emptying their bladders. The stagnation causes smoldering infection, and that makes them wet the bed."

"I hadn't even thought of anything like that," Clarice said.

"Then there are the sound sleepers," I went on. "Boys who just don't wake up until after it's too late. We can usually help them get over bedwetting pretty easily, and of course it isn't their fault that they sleep soundly."

"George sleeps like a rock, all right. In fact, even when you get him up and walk him to the bathroom, he doesn't remember a thing about it in the morning."

"Let's try the conditioned reflex system for a little while, then, and see whether we can tie the act of voiding a little more tightly to the bathroom."

When the Russian scientist Pavlov rang a bell each time he fed his dogs, he found later that he could make them slobber just by ringing the bell. You can use the same action as a training aid, although I think it is more pleasant to use a little music box rather than a bell. If the child turns on a music box every time he gets ready to void in the daytime, he will link that sound and the bathroom surroundings with the act of urination. After a few weeks of this, he will have sound, spot and action linked together in his mind. If you get him up just before you go to bed, take him to the bathroom, and start the music box playing, he will usually void quite readily. After a few weeks of nightly emptying, he will often reach a point where he gets up without aid instead of wetting the bed.

7

Time-Tested Remedies for Sexual and Menopausal Complaints

Sexual afflictions are triply disturbing. They make you miserable, they frequently lead to embarrassment, and they undermine your sexual self-confidence. Why suffer messy discharge, embarrassing itch, sexually debilitating congestion, and menopausal miseries? Home care can help you with all of these conditions and many others.

HOW TO CONTROL FEMALE TROUBLES WITH HOME MEASURES

Mild or moderate discharge, itching, and irritation of the female outlet frequently yield to simple home measures. Profuse watery discharge usually deserves a doctor's care, especially if it causes a great deal of itching burning or surface rawness. So does thick, whitish discharge accompanied by severe itching which is often due to fungus infection. Women in their sixties and seventies, who often suffer from a special form of vaginal irritation and discharge which yields promptly to female sex hormones, can get worthwhile help from a doctor. If you decide that prescription measures might help you, always take a sanitary belt and several pads to the doctor's office with you, since some of the medicines used stain clothing irreparably.

Whitish discharge. Ordinary whitish discharge usually yields to vinegar douching, which you can manage quite well at home.

Vinegar douches. Plain vinegar restores vaginal acidity and clears up most cases of simple discharge. Use an ordinary douche bag with a hard rubber tip. Make up the douche solution with four tablespoonfuls of white vinegar and two quarts of warm water. Lubricate the douche tip with petroleum or lubricating jelly, and insert it. Hold the lips of the female organ snugly together around the base of the tip, and start the solution running in with the bag a foot or two above the douche tip opening. When water pressure balloons out the organ and opens up all the deep wrinkles and creases, you will feel a slight stretching sensation. Release the lips of the female organ and let the douche fluid flow freely for a moment while the vagina collapses into folds again. Repeat this process several times, until the douche fluid is exhausted. Most victims of ordinary discharge need to douche daily for about ten days and two to three times weekly thereafter.

How to control itching at the female opening. Itching of the female opening without excessive discharge often yields to home measures. Try this program:

First two days: Cleanse the area twice daily with a mild detergent such as pHisoderm and several cotton balls. Four times daily, mix one table-spoonful of Burow's solution with one cup of water and use to wet a washcloth or piece of cotton. Place this against the itching area for ten minutes. Or use Tucks, which are medicated pads obtainable without a prescription. They contain the same active ingredient as Burow's.

Until itching is completely controlled (usually about one week): Get one ounce of Lassar's paste from your druggist (no prescription required). Dry thoroughly after each cleansing and apply a thin coat of the paste.

After itching ceases: Continue cleansing once a day. Dry thoroughly. Powder lightly with cornstarch. Continue this program for two weeks.

Your doctor can give worthwhile help if itching does not yield promptly to this program or if it is accompanied by excessive discharge, a lump, or a sore or leathery white patch.

HOME MANAGEMENT OF MASTURBATION

"I just know he's playing with himself," Gloria said. "I'll find stiff soiled handkerchiefs around, and sometimes dirty pictures. But he doesn't have a father you know, and I just can't bring myself to talk about it."

Gloria's son was a well-developed fifteen, old enough to have sired a child or two when humankind hid out in caves and bushes, but still a mere boy according to our present lights. Hormones change a few eons less quickly than civilization's customs, though, and the boy had all the glandular functions of a grown and married man.

"I'll talk to him if you want," I said. "But I'm probably not going to say what you expect."

Reassurance. "I'll tell him just what my old professor used to say: ninety percent of boys admit to masturbation and the other ten percent are liars. I know that some churches regard it as a sin, and I'll make it clear to him that the rights and wrongs of masturbation aren't entirely based on medical facts. But I'll try to set him straight on any old wives' tales he's heard about masturbation stunting his growth or affecting his mind and any confusion he might have of masturbation and homosexuality.''

Masturbation injury. Physical injury from masturbation is not a problem with boys, but girls (over half of whom also use some form of sexual self-stimulation) sometimes have difficulties. When a girl complains of whitish, irritating discharge, she often has a small object or a piece of an object up inside the vagina. If you can approach the subject in a way which does not seem harshly critical or accusatory, she will often tell you what has happened. In most cases, these objects can readily be removed without medical instruments. Bleeding sometimes comes from a torn virginal membrane. If you spread the folds so that you can see where the bleeder is spurting, firm pressure from a cotton ball for five minutes by the clock (without any interruption for peeks to see whether the treatment is working) will usually stop the flow. In these situations, and also in those requiring medical care, it is important to approach the problem in a matter-of-fact, noncritical manner—shame and embarrassment are great strains to the young mind, and often interfere with later sexual adjustment. Why add these burdens to the already substantial adjustment problems of youth?

Undue sexual curiosity. Many years ago, a six-year-old boy was brought to me because he ''took down the neighbor's young girl's panties.''

''It's natural and normal for a six-year-old to want to know more about the difference between boys and girls,'' I said. ''He could probably have picked a way that wouldn't offend neighborhood manners and morals, but there's nothing wrong with his mind or his sexual development.''

''Then we shouldn't do anything about it?'' the boy's parents asked.

''Have a little talk with him, if you can do it without getting embarrassed or upset, but aim at assuaging his curiosity instead of condemning his behavior. Show him pictures, explain how the male and female organs fit together. If you can feel totally comfortable about it, you might let down the modesty barriers a bit around the house. Perhaps you can work on the assumption that the sight of your private parts is something which should be reserved for members of the family, but needn't be restricted particularly within the home.''

I dug back into ancient history for this case because I know how that youngster turned out: he's a respected minister, happily married and father of three children. He has never been involved in any sexual impropriety since then, in spite of (or more likely because of) his parents' tolerant, noncritical response to this incident.

HOW TO CONTROL COMMON MALE SEX MISERIES WITH HOME MEASURES

You can avoid or quickly cure penile irritations, urethritis, and some prostate troubles with home measures. Cleansing methods, contraceptive or hygienic measures, sex habits, and fluid balance all enter into your program for controlling sex organ difficulties. Medicines and special supplies are seldom required.

Crab lice. Most victims pick up crab lice from public toilets, not by sex contact. Look for the little devils whenever you get much itching down below. They are brownish in color and almost half as big as an ordinary wood tick. Sometimes you can spot the pearly gray eggs adhering to pubic hairs more easily than the burrowing lice.

Ointment. I usually suggest Kwell ointment for crab lice. Apply to the crotch, pubic hair area, and armpits twice a day for two days.

DDT. Ten per cent DDT powder is cheaper than ointment, and is quite effective in most cases. Apply two or three times a day for three days.

Shave, trim or comb. With DDT powder and other methods aimed at the adult lice only, you need to shave the whole area gently but thoroughly or go over it with a fine toothed comb. The fine toothed comb works best if you have applied towels wet with vinegar solution (two tablespoonfuls to a pint of warm water) for 20 minutes. Since the recommended ointment kills eggs as well as lice, you can trim the hairs to half inch length with this method instead of shaving or combing, and avoid considerable discomfort.

Laundry precautions. Home laundry or laundromat machines do not use hot enough water to kill crabs. Best send underclothing to a commercial laundry or boil it for ten minutes.

Crotch itch. Another common condition spread through locker room benches and the like is crotch or jock-strap itch. This is a distant cousin of athlete's foot, caused by the same family of microbes. It shows up as dusky red patches on the inner sides of both upper thighs, sometimes with slight scaling. Undecenylic acid ointment (Desenex) twice a day for a week usually effects a cure.

Penile irritations. A sore on the penis within eight weeks after random sexual contact deserves prompt medical care. Likewise any sore or lump which does not heal promptly with home measures. However, most penile irritations yield quickly to simple home care.

Smegma irritation. Instead of ordinary skin oil, the glands inside the foreskin make a thick, smelly, whitish material. When the tip of the penis or foreskin becomes raw, irritation from this smegma is often at fault.

Thorough cleansing. Smegma irritation usually clears up promptly if you cleanse thoroughly beneath the foreskin every day for a week. Prevent recurrences by cleansing once a week. During a warm bath, strip back the foreskin and wash away any accumulated whitish matter. If the foreskin is tight, be sure to pull it forward again immediately after cleansing: otherwise, the squeeze it makes on the penis may cause enough swelling to make replacement painful or difficult.

Glycerin. A few men find that their smegma is particularly difficult to remove with soap and water. They get relief with a little glycerin applied with cotton, then wiped off five to ten minutes later with a washrag or clean cloth.

Irritation after intercourse. Itchy, burning swellings of the penis within 24 hours after intercourse are usually due to contraceptive or feminine hygiene preparations which your wife is using. A change in brands of birth control materials and replacement of fancy douche powders with ordinary vinegar usually gives quick cure.

Occasionally, I see a patient with swelling and soreness on the under side of the tip of the penis, where a slim band of tissue attaches the foreskin to the head of the penis itself. This almost always stems from excessive sexual friction. Lubrication with lubricating or petroleum jelly during sexual relations usually prevents further difficulty, and aids sexual satisfaction, too.

Genital herpes. Since the previous edition of this book, a new form of genital irritation has become very common all over the world. The virus that has always caused fever blisters has undergone a change in its makeup, and now frequently affects the penis and vagina. This condition first came to light in patients whose ability to fight off infections had been impaired by strong drugs, such as those given to fight cancer. Viruses which learned to survive in human tissue under these circumstances then spread to otherwise healthy men and women.

The sores of genital herpes look and act very much like the old familiar fever blister, starting with an irregular-shaped watery blob surrounded by an area of redness and inflammation. If you identify it at this stage, there is no confusion whatever with syphilis or other more serious diseases, which produce a thickened sore with a punched-out ulcer in the middle. Herpes also sends many unhappy signals of its presence in the form of pain and tenderness: most of my patients find that it makes sexual intercourse almost impossible because of sharp burning pain with stretching or exposure to sexual secretions. After the blister breaks, a thin crust forms over the sore, and pain becomes slightly less intense. Each individual sore usually smoulders along for about three weeks before it heals, with a further crop often arising before the first one is healed. Genital herpes shows up much more readily in men than in women because the sores are always on the surface. In women, sores often are located within the vagina (although they also occur on the inner lips).

If you identify a new sore inside a few hours of onset, you may be able to stop it with silver nitrate solution. Pass a needle (not a pin) through the flame of a match to sterilize it, and be sure that it does not touch any nonsterile surface after flaming until use. Clean off the top of the sore with rubbing alcohol (which will sting a bit). Unroof the blister with the needle, which you will find relatively painless because the layer of skin that forms the top of the blister has no nerve supply. Apply silver nitrate solution with the end of a match or with a very small cotton tipped applicator. As soon as the surface of the sore turns white, neutralize the silver nitrate with a thorough alcohol wash. This treatment converts the smouldering virus infection (often lasting for weeks) into a small, clean slough which generally heals in about two days.

After the first few hours, or if the blister has already broken and formed a scab, silver nitrate will not work. At this stage your best bet is hydrocortisone cream, recently made available on a nonprescription basis. Hydrocortisone cream is expensive, and only the layer in actual contact with the sore does any good, so you can make a tube go a lot farther by putting a tiny dab in the center of the sore and waiting until it warms to your skin for a minute or so before spreading it with a wooden matchstick or the like.

Recent studies have shown that you heal herpes sores much more quickly and make any recurrent sores milder by raising your body's supply of zinc. I usually use a preparation called Vi Con C for this purpose, which contains both zinc and other nutrients which affect tissue healing. Other forms of zinc obtainable in nutrition centers work equally well, if you can get your intake up to about 80 mcg per day. The label usually identifies strength in terms of mcgs, so you can take as many tablets as are required to add up to an appropriate dose.

Irritation from harsh chemicals. Itching and rash on the shaft of the penis usually is due to chemicals or irritants you handle or get on your clothing during the day, transferred to the penis during urination. Cutting oils and chemicals which will not irritate the thick skin of your fingers often make the delicate skin of the penis raw. Solution: Wash your hands thoroughly before urinating, and drop soiled work trousers instead of using the fly. If this fails (as with one of my patients, who ultimately proved allergic to the soap supplied at his working place!), handle the organ through several layers of a clean handkerchief when you need to void during working hours.

How to control urethritis. Although any whitish discharge or burning on urination should send you to your doctor immediately if you have had sexual contact with a possibly infected woman inside of two weeks, many infections of the urethra occur without any possibility of venereal disease. In these cases, prompt home measures at the first sign of burning or discharge often lead to cure.

Flooding with fluid. If you drink four to five quarts of water, ginger ale, or fruit juice a day for two to three days starting immediately after the first twinge of burning, you can frequently flush out the urethra thoroughly enough to control the attack.

After-sex urination. If you are subject to nonvenereal infection of the tube from the bladder to the exterior, empty your bladder soon after intercourse. This condition commonly occurs when the germs from the body surface manage to get up into the more delicate portions of the urethra. These germs cannot grow in or swim along the fast-moving urinary stream, but they can grow along or swim up through the protein-rich moisture left behind by sexual excitement or intercourse. Prompt urination usually washes away any residue of protein-rich fluid before germs have a chance to multiply in it and cause an infection.

What about "morning pearl"? After a long period of abstinence from sex, many men begin to find a drop or two of thick white matter at the penile opening every morning. This so-called morning pearl is usually due to very mild nonvenereal infection or to simple overflow of sex gland secretion. If sexual relief is not possible, flushing the passage by means of high fluid intake usually brings relief.

Prostate congestion. Impaired potency, low backache and tiredness usually point toward congestion or infection of the prostate gland. While severe cases call for a doctor's care, you can often restore potency and gain comfort in mild cases with home measures.

Hot sitz baths. Put four inches of hot water (112 degrees) in your bathtub. Sit in it for 20 minutes, adding more hot water as necessary to maintain the temperature. If you do not have an accurate thermometer, test the water with your hand when adding hot water to insure against burns. Wrap a towel around your shoulders during the sitz bath to keep from getting chilled.

Scrotal dip. Although hot sitz baths often help to relieve the congestion that leads to sagging potency, the heat tends to soothe sexual excitement to a degree. If you plan prompt sexual exercise, you may find a ten to thirty second dip of the scrotal contents in very cold water helpful. Ice water in an ordinary tumbler works quite well in restoring excitability.

Prostate infection. You usually get worthwhile help from your doctor if you are suffering from actual prostate infection. Extreme impairment of potency, backache, burning on urination, and sometimes slight discharge point toward this condition. One helpful home test is the three glass procedure: pass a few drops of urine in one glass, almost all of what remains in another glass, and the last teaspoonful in a third. Cloudiness in the first glass only usually points to urethritis, while cloudiness in both the first and the third glass almost always means prostate infection.

Prostate disorder proneness. If you have had several spells of prostatitis or if you have smoldering, nonvenereal urethritis, you should rigorously avoid jolting and vibration. A rough ride in a truck or tractor milks material in and out of the prostate gland. If any germs have worked their way back along the urethra to the prostate's opening, which is just below the bladder, the prostate gland becomes infected. The steps we already discussed for avoiding urethritis obviously help to keep germs away from the prostate opening, and thus make jolting and vibration less dangerous. A hydraulic seat or several layers of foam rubber padding help to make vibrating machinery, trucks or tractors less hazardous. A high intake of fluids during working hours makes for more frequent voiding, which flushes germs away from the prostate opening.

Prostate enlargement. When the prostate gland enlarges, it pushes up into the tube from the bladder to the outside. While the prostate seldom blocks the urethra completely, it often prevents the bladder from entirely emptying itself. When your prostate gland enlarges, you may notice some difficulty in starting to urinate. The urinary stream may become less forceful. A sense of not completely emptying the bladder is common. Since the bladder does not empty completely, it fills again more quickly than before: frequent voiding during the day and two or more trips to the toilet at night become necessary. If the condition gets no care, infection usually occurs, causing burning, fever, and extreme frequency. The enlarged gland may block the urinary passage entirely, making the bladder expand painfully.

Hot packs. As a temporary measure of relief, you can often get the urinary stream started by applying hot towels to the crotch and lower abdomen. Change the towels frequently. Usually, it is wise to let a small stream of water run from the tap, too: the sound of running water often helps to relieve tension in the urinary muscles.

Whenever prostate enlargement makes special measures necessary to start the stream, you can definitely get worthwhile help from your doctor. Most such trouble is due to a disorder which never causes cancer. Your doctor can arrange to have the portion of the gland which is blocking the urinary passage pared back electrically, thus avoiding all need for a cutting operation.

HOW TO EASE YOUR WAY THROUGH THE MENOPAUSE

The menopause! How often have you heard that word uttered with a fearful shudder? Until modern science learned to prevent or relieve the miseries of the menopause, many people suffered grave distress. Sex organs became a source of botheration and distress to most women and to many men. Today, you can prevent or quickly cure every affliction the menopause might bring. You can keep your sex life satisfying for many years beyond. You can solve most menopause-period sex problems for yourself, right in your own home.

About half of the women and one-fourth of the men in America need help from a doctor for menopausal complaints at one time or another. The problems which yield most readily to prescription-type hormones are hot flashes, sinking spells, abrupt sweating spells, periods of mental fogginess, and creeping, crawling skin sensations. If you suffer from such complaints, a few tablets usually give tremendous help. There is no need to hold back because of fear that you will become more needful of hormones because of what you take. Hormone tablets work to cushion the shock of abrupt change in your body's natural hormone levels. You can usually cut your dose in half within six months and taper to no tablets at all within two years.

Incidentally, tablets work just as well as shots. Thousands of men and women pay needlessly large sums for help with the menopause because of the unwarranted idea that shots are better than pills. The hormone gets into your bloodstream before it has any effect, and it gets there just as reliably from your stomach as from your hip.

Fight menopausal blues with this philosophy. Most of my patients have found one measure even more helpful than hormones in fighting menopausal miseries: developing a different viewpoint toward this period of life. The menopause is not the end of something. It is the beginning of your period of reward: the period when the effort you have put into raising a family begins to justify itself in their success, when your skills and interests bear top fruit, when the home you struggled to build up and keep is all your own. Nothing stops with the menopause, except the inconvenience of monthly bleeding. Sex continues, love continues, strength and skill remain unchanged. That simple fact sometimes affords relief from the blue feelings many people name as the menopause's most stringent plague.

How to enjoy sex after the menopause. A great many women are surprised to find that sex either remains just as enjoyable or becomes considerably more so after the menopause. Until the menopause, the possibility of pregnancy hangs heavily over every couple's sex life. A woman is never unconcerned about fertility: either she wants babies or she doesn't. She can't indulge in sex for love and pleasure alone as long as pregnancy might possibly result.

After the menopause, neither *hope for* nor *fear of* pregnancy interferes. Both husband and wife can cast off many grave concerns and uncertainties. Each can pursue sex for his own and his partner's satisfaction with concentration and skill never before possible.

How to develop your sexual skill. Selfish sex is always a failure. That's why sexual skill always aims at satisfying the other person. Your partner's response then increases your pleasure and satisfaction. Here are three pointers about married sex which most couples find worthwhile:

Preen for your partner. By age thirty-five or so, many husbands and wives unwittingly begin to take their marriage partners for granted sexually. They pass up simple ways of making themselves more attractive. They don't take time to preen. A little more effort devoted to evening showers, shaves, toothbrushing, perfume, negligee and other bedtime grooming (not to mention avoiding negatives like face cream, curlers and such) often makes more difference than the best-planned erotic campaign.

Keep variety in your caresses. It's wonderful to know what your sex partner likes, and to put that knowledge to work. But if you could sit down right now and write the exact caresses your husband or wife will expect the next time you have sex, variety could add new heights of excitement to your marriage bed. Change the order of your approach. Change the type of caress from stroke to grasp, from kiss to gentle nip, from rhythmic rub to vibrating tickle. Give special care to the last stage of your sex play: full passionate preparation calls for culmination caresses which should never seem routine.

Gain new thrills or greater ease and comfort through different sex positions. A husband and wife can fit together sexually in literally dozens of ways. The standard position has one advantage: both husband and wife can contribute what they wish with caresses, loving words, and activity. Certain other positions help keep your sexual attraction ever fresh by adding variety. Still others meet certain frequent health or sexual needs.

Here are the most important special approaches:

Important nerve centers come into play with the wife in a bent-knees, bent hips posture, especially after you reach full-blown maturity. Through the years of marriage, sex sensitivity gradually shifts in the female organ. Spots toward the front far up inside the female organ become keener. The husband can often please and satisfy a mature wife much more thoroughly if he directs his thrust forward. To do this, he brings his wife's knees up beside his chest with her hips folded.

Any long-married couple can vary their sex life through the wife's-heels-on-husband's shoulders position. They begin intercourse in standard position. After contact, the wife stretches her legs straight up. The husband rears back slightly, and moves his arms one at a time to a position outside his wife's legs. The wife then hooks the back of her heels on his shoulders. The husband contributes all sexual activity from then on, although his wife can respond freely with words and caresses.

Make your union snugger with the wife's-legs-straight position. A woman who has borne several children may have a stretched, over-spacious vagina. This makes it hard for her to satisfy her husband. But if she keeps her legs straight down and her husband spreads his legs to straddle hers, both partners can reach a keen climax.

Enjoy sex without exertion with the postero-lateral or the crossed approach. Both these positions allow moderate sexual satisfaction when illness or loss of strength makes vigorous approach difficult. For the postero-lateral approach, both partners lie on their right sides. The husband approaches from the rear while the wife keeps her hips and knees bent. The crossed position finds the wife lying on her back with hips folded. The husband lies on his right side crosswise on the bed.

8

Modified Remedies for Colds, Sore Throats, and Coughs

Of all the miseries to which you fall heir, the one you most frequently have to fight off for yourself is the common cold. You have probably resigned yourself to these miseries in the past. "Nothing really helps," people have told you. "A cold lasts a week if you dose yourself up, and seven days if you don't."

The picture need not be that grim. Look at these practical, effective measures, which you can take right in your own home.

SPEED COLD RECOVERY WITH SIMPLE MEANS

Shorten colds with better drainage. Your body has a very effective way of fighting off any germs that try to gain a foothold within its tissues. Thousands of germ-devouring white blood cells get to the scene in a matter of moments. Each of these cells stuffs itself with germs. As long as there is some place for the stuffed, useless white blood cells to go, your body washes them away on a wave of fluid and sends other germ-devouring white blood cells in their place.

That's why good drainage helps your nose and sinuses. A cold makes your nose lining swell and closes off pockets of infection. If you shrink your swollen nose lining with proper medication, trapped pus can drain away. A new horde of white blood cells can get to work, throwing off your infection.

Nose lining shrinkers. Although I recommended nose drops and sprays in previous editions of this book, the newer nose lining shrinkers have almost made them obsolete. My first choice is Sudafed, which contains the most effective congestion-relieving agent without a lot of other junk thrown in. Most cold victims don't need the antihistamines (which may cause drowsiness) or secretion-driers (which make the remaining secretions thicker and more adherent) contained in Contac, Dristan, Actifed and other cold remedy mixtures. These mixed-formula pills or capsules do have a place for people with an extensive background of allergy, whose colds often stir up dormant allergic disease. Without an allergic background, though, you're probably better off with the straight stuff. Sudafed sold on a nonprescription basis has about half the strength of the prescription type medicines, but there's a simple answer to that: if one pill doesn't give relief, take two at a time. Two every eight hours should be the limit, though. If you haven't obtained relief with that dose, more won't help.

This is a good time to emphasize the importance of reading the fine print on medicine labels. All cold pills, including Sudafed, have a strong warning on the label regarding use by people with high blood pressure, heart disease, and in some instances pregnancy. Yet I still see dozens of people every month who have taken these preparations when the directions plainly say that they should not.

So what should they do? If the label on the cold pills and capsules says that a person in your condition should not take them, old-fashioned nose drops become your best bet. Sparing use of ¼% Neosynephrine is safe for all but a handful of the most severe blood pressure or heart disease victims (who should check with their doctor with every cold anyway). Squirt one puff into each nostril, straight up the nose passage toward the center of your forehead, with an atomizer. Wait ten minutes, then repeat *once* if necessary. Or lie on your back with your head hanging over the edge of the bed, turn your chin toward your right shoulder and put two drops in the right nostril. Let them soak in for 30 seconds, then turn to the left and do the left nostril. Use nose drops every three or four hours if necessary for two or three days, but never continue their use for more than three days at a time. Continued use of nose drops often leads to rebound congestion—stuffiness four or five hours after the application which actually comes from reaction to the drops themselves. I have seen patients who remained stopped up for months simply because "the only way I can breathe is to take more drops." This miserable vicious circle is the main reason for limiting drops to people who can't use anything else, but you can avoid the problem by keeping your period of nose drop use down to two or three days with each cold.

Soothing spray or snuffling solution. After the first three to seven days of a cold, most nasal stuffiness and sinus blockage is usually due to thick mucus instead of swollen nose lining. At this point you should stop using lining shrinkers or drops. You usually can get a great deal of relief by thinning the thick material. Easy techniques: Either spray or snuff up a soothing, mucus-thinning solution into your nose. Use this recipe:

> 1 level teaspoonful table salt.
> 1 pint distilled water.
> 2–4 drops Eau de Cologne if desired for pleasant scent.

If you do not have distilled water, you can use tap water by letting it stand overnight in a shallow pan to allow the chlorine to escape. Use with an atomizer, or pour a couple of teaspoonfuls into the hollow of your hand and snuff it up. One such spraying or snuffing every three to four hours usually keeps the passages open.

Get better more quickly, more safely, and more cheaply by holding antibiotics in reserve. Penicillin works wonders against germs it can attack. It is absolutely worthless for anything caused by a virus, particularly colds, flu, and ordinary sore throats. Four out of five doses of penicillin given for colds or sore throats are actually worthless or harmful. If you hold penicillin and other germ killers in reserve, you will avoid many serious drug allergies. You will get more effective care for complications such as ear or sinus infections, which are just as frequent and much more stubborn when penicillin is used for the original cold. And you will save money.

How can you hold penicillin in reserve? Don't take penicillin on your own, either by buying a supply without a doctor's prescription or by starting on left-over medicine from a previous illness. Take care of milder colds and sore throats for yourself, with the measures described in this chapter. If a severe cold drives you to your doctor, tell him that you'll be especially pleased if he can get you through without using germ killers. And don't go to a doctor who prescribes germ killers without a careful examination and a blood count. A doctor who decides that you need penicillin after one look at your nose and throat isn't giving you scientific treatment: he's playing a lazy man's guessing game.

Make colds briefer, avoid sinus trouble, and keep your hearing sharper by controlled nose blowing. Want to cut your colds to only three days each, even if they've been averaging two weeks or longer? That's what a young Air Force doctor did for his charges during World War II. The main feature of his cold program didn't require any complicated steps: it was to cut down nose blowing.

Your nose is always loaded with dangerous germs. Some of the spaces with which it is linked, the sinuses and the cavities of the ears, normally have no germs in them at all. Sweeper cells guard the entrances to these spaces, but sweep only at a very slow rate. They can't keep ahead of a burst of air pushed by a cough or a sneeze. They can't keep ahead of the blast you make whenever you blow your nose.

That's why you can cut the length of your colds, cut your chance of getting sinus trouble, and decrease the biggest single danger to your sharp hearing by taking a single step: throw away your handkerchief and try to forget nose-blowing!

The habit of a lifetime is hard to break. Sniff and swallow. Wipe your nose gently. But if you find yourself blowing before you know it, blow gently with both nostrils open. Never stop up the free nostril to blast open the closed-over one. Settle for one breathing space if you must, but don't blast yourself into a miserable sinus infection.

Rest to build up your resistance. The fastest way to beat a cold is undoubtedly in bed. Second best is a day broken with rest intervals: at least one half-hour rest at lunch time or before supper, plus ten hours in bed at night.

Aspirin or Tylenol. If aches and pains disturb your rest, take two aspirin or Tylenol tablets after each meal and at bedtime whether you feel as if you need them or not. Take these medications by the day, not by the ache: on and off dosage sometimes kicks your fever curve up and down, making for extra sweats and chilly sensations. This amount of aspirin is perfectly safe. The after-meals timing almost always prevents nausea. Take aspirin or Tylenol regularly throughout the cold, until aches and pains have thoroughly subsided.

Although aspirin is the old reliable, I have switched most of my patients to Tylenol. Aspirin on an empty stomach almost always causes a bit of irritation in the stomach lining. In fact, there is small but measurable blood loss through the bowel in almost everyone who takes aspirin. This problem can be kept to a tolerable minimum by taking aspirin after meals or with milk, but cold victims often need relief between meals or when they haven't any appetite. Tylenol seems equally effective for this use (although not for some other applications, such as relief of joint pain) without the keep-it-after-meals bother.

Dodge he-man germs during a cold. One person in five who starts with an ordinary cold or sore throat gets some further infection before he gets well. A cold weakens your body's defenses so that you get sick from germs which you could ordinarily fight off with ease. But here's a hopeful fact: the germs that cause serious infections are seldom in your nose or throat when the original cold strikes. *If you can dodge new germ families for the first few days of a cold, you can cut your chance of sinus or chest infection at least in half.*

How can you dodge new germ families? Fortunately, most of them actually come from other members of your family or circle of friends. You can cut your germ exposure tremendously by taking three simple steps:

1. Avoid germ-laden mouth moisture. Sanitation will never make mankind give up the kiss. But why not refrain during colds, and shift to the cheek when in doubt? Why share one bathroom glass with the whole household? Small plastic glasses cost only a few cents apiece. One for each member of your family, perhaps colored to match his toothbrush, will take up very little space. Likewise with mouth-touching toys, food from other people's plates and so on.

2. *Spray-rinse dishes and let them drain dry.* The best germ-dodging policy actually saves work here! Dishes are much more free of germs if they are sprayed or rinsed with very hot water and left to dry than if you work them over with a towel.

3. *Use space to prevent germ spread.* Most of the germs which people spread into the air when they talk are in relatively large droplets. These fall to the ground within six feet. Chairs arranged so the people's heads are six feet apart let many less germs pass from person to person in your living room, dining room, and office or shop.

These three steps—avoiding mouth moisture, spray-rinsing dishes, and keeping at moderate distance—keep down the number of excess germs you face while a cold is cutting down your body's power to fight.

Children's Dosages

You can calculate the proper dosage for most medicines, including aspirin and cough preparations, by following the table devised at Guy's Hospital, London. To use this table, first determine the safe adult dose from package literature or label. BE VERY CAREFUL TO DISTINGUISH "GRAINS" (ABBREVIATED GR.) FROM "GRAMS" (ABBREVIATED GM.) WHICH ARE FIFTEEN TIMES AS LARGE. Determine the content of a child's size tablet or the strength of a teaspoonful (one dram or 5 cc) of liquid, and figure from there.

Age	Fraction of Adult Dose	Age	Fraction of Adult Dose
1 month	1/20	3 years	1/5
3 months	1/15	4 years	1/4
6 months	1/10	5 & 6 years	1/3
9 months	1/9	7 & 8 years	1/2
1 year	1/7	10 to 12 years	2/3
2 years	1/6	13 to 15 years	3/4

HOW TO FIGHT COLD-PRONENESS

Almost anyone can substantially reduce his exposure to cold germs and substantially increase his resistance to them. If you are particularly subject to colds, home measures to counteract this tendency usually prove especially worthwhile. These measures are more effective than any cold shot yet devised, and involve absolutely no medical expense or risk.

You cannot dodge cold germs simply by avoiding people who sneeze and cough. Colds spread mainly before complaints begin, and reach you mainly from members of your own family or close circle of friends. A few germs, even of the worst possible kind, do you no harm. It takes thousands or millions of germs, all from the same germ family, to set up disease. Even one less than the crucial number leads to no trouble at all. You can cut down spread of germs through mouth moisture, improperly sanitized dishes, and close quarters in the firm knowledge that even a few less germs spread may mean a great deal less sickness in your household.

Protect your nose lining against cold germs. Some home measures for preventing colds are just common sense: enough rest, well-chosen foods, and sufficient warm clothing. Science can add two tremendous aids: extra help for your body's main shield against cold germs, which is your nose lining, and heightened resistance through cold-fighting morale.

How your nose lining protects you against germs. Your nose lining spreads an invisibly thin sheet of sticky mucus over the entire inside of your nose. When you breathe in germs, most of them stick in the sheet of mucus. Tiny sweeper cells continually brush the mucus back into your throat. A brand new sheet forms every six minutes or so. Meanwhile sweepings pile up at the back of your throat until they make a glob big enough for you to swallow. Your stomach acids kill the germs.

In the wintertime, the dry, heated air turns your nose lining's mucus blanket to crusts. It may even dry the nose lining until it cracks, providing completely free access to germs. Moisturization prevents this effect, and thus increases your nose lining's resistance.

How can you moisturize your nose lining? Three main methods are worthwhile:

1. Add moisture to heated air. Humidifiers or moisturizing pans on the radiators are worthwhile. They at least take the edge off the dryness of indoor air. They cannot do the whole job, since thorough home air moisturization requires evaporation of several gallons of water each day.

2. Turn down the heat. When you warm air from 58 degrees to 80 degrees, you increase its drying power more than eightfold. It's best to heat your house only to 60 degrees or so and put on extra sweaters or heavier clothes for bodily warmth. At night, you can cool your bedroom five or ten degrees by turning heat down or by ventilation. That gives your nose lining a rest from too-dry, overheated air. An extra comforter or an electric blanket keeps your body warm.

3. Use home-made moisturizing nose spray. You can banish dry crusts and help your nose's defense by using this moisturizing spray:

1 tablespoonful glycerin, obtained from any drugstore
   without prescription.
1½ tablespoonfuls 70% alcohol (rubbing alcohol strength).
1 teaspoonful table salt.
1 pint tap or distilled water.

If your tap water has a heavy odor of chlorine, let it stand overnight in an open vessel. Mix the ingredients and stir until salt is thoroughly dissolved. Pour into clean bottle and stopper firmly.

Get a plastic pocket atomizer for about a dollar at the drugstore, fill it with this solution, and use it several times a day as needed.

Last-minute action to ward off a cold. Can you tell when a cold is just coming on? If you can, you may be able to stop some colds from getting a real start.

The first thing to try is moisturizing spray (see above). Spray the inside of your nose thoroughly every hour or two. Keep warm and get a good night's sleep. This program alone will stop some colds in their tracks.

If you have enough colds to make it worthwhile, one other medicine might help you. It's a combination of codeine and papaverine, which are available on prescription only. When used at the first sign of a cold, it sometimes stops the nose lining responses which allow germs to get a foothold. When you next see your doctor, ask him if you should have this material on hand and how you should use it when you feel a cold coming on.

Vitamin C keeps cropping up as a cold-fighting aid. Years ago, it was very popular in 25–50 mgm doses "at the first sign of a cold." Studies with similar-looking sugar pills showed no real effect from this dosage. Under its new name of "ascorbic acid" Vitamin C has recently been advised in doses of 250–500 mgms "when you first feel a cold coming on." Some world-recognized experts have given this dosage their support, but I haven't seen any definite proof. The trouble is that everyone thinks he's going to get a cold several times as often as he actually gets one, so studies done without the sugar pill routine are subject to error. Vitamin C won't hurt you, though, if you want to give it a try.

Fight colds by mental measures. Parts of your brain actually govern your circulation and many other bodily functions through which you fight off germs. Your emotional state greatly influences these functions. It can thus help or hurt your resistance to all kinds of infection. This effect is very strong. Just thinking you are liable to get a cold may tip the balance and make you fall victim to one.

A research expert proved the importance of emotions in the origin of colds without even trying. He wanted to grow cold germs in the laboratory. In order to tell whether the germs were present in his culture solution, he decided to spray some into a few people's noses. The subjects were kept in hospital rooms and protected from new infections until any strong germs they already had acquired would have shown up. (Some cold germs are probably present in most people's throats all the time, but not enough to cause a cold so long as their resistance is normal.) Then he sprayed a few people with ordinary water, telling them the stuff was loaded with germs. One out of five promptly came down with a cold.

The rest of the experiment proved that strong cold germs were present in the doctor's other mixture. But this very first step proved a point which is very important to you. It means that even weak cold germs can be helped along by mental forces until they overcome your resistance. When you get chilled or feel a draught, the chances are that you say to yourself: "Now I'm in for it! I'll have a cold tomorrow for sure!" That conviction itself causes concern and emotional response which actually help to give you the cold.

Build your cold-fighting morale. You can protect yourself against two thirds of all colds by building cold-fighting morale. That's what a team of researchers at Michigan found when they were experimenting with a new cold vaccine. They thought they had an effective product, and designed tests to prove the fact. One group of people got the vaccine. Another group got nothing, and still another got distilled water, being told that they were getting cold shots.

When the results were in, the people who took the cold shots reported only one third as many colds as the ones who had nothing at all. But the ones who got the distilled water had even less! The conviction that they would get less colds actually cut the number of colds these people suffered tremendously!

What does this mean to you? Certainly not that your colds aren't real: they're real, germ-caused infections. But your resistance may be affected so much by concern about old wives' tales that you have many colds which you would otherwise fight off.

This need not be. You can use mental forces to *increase* your resistance instead of impair it. You can build your cold-fighting morale to the point where you have many less colds per year.

How to build cold-fighting morale. Cold-fighting morale is best built on one firm conviction: *nothing that happens to you can give you a cold.*

You need never say to yourself: "Drat it! I did thus-and-so, so now I'll probably get a cold!" Absolutely none of the common experiences you might note can give you a cold.

Let's look at some of the ideas science has explored in reaching this conclusion:

Draughts, night air, and going without a hat do not cause colds. The lining of your nose is definitely affected by nerve and emotional balance. Your nose can get stopped up or runny on the basis of pure nerve reflex when you are exposed to wind or cold. It can get stopped up and runny after any uncomfortable nerve-tickling exposure, even through slight draughts. But unless worry or concern add further burdens, your nose lining will usually get back to normal before the ever-present cold germs actually get a start.

Chilling doesn't cause colds. When I was only a child, I remember my aunt stomping her feet one day as she came in the front door.

"Brrr—" she said. "I'm chilled clean through. Have a cold tomorrow, like as not."

The next day, sure enough! She had a cold. But today's science says that my aunt probably already had the cold germs in her body, and those germs were already starting disease when she first walked in my door and said "Brrr—." My aunt almost certainly felt chilly because of a beginning cold; she didn't get the cold because of the chill. But millions of people are positive that whenever they get chilled, a cold will certainly follow. If they actually do get chilled, not simply get chilly sensations because of a beginning cold, how many of them actually suffer a cold, not because of the chill, but because of fearful certainty that they are headed for the sickbed?

Have confidence in your body's powers. Of course, it pays to dress yourself warmly and to avoid extreme exposure. But it pays to have confidence in your body, too. Take reasonable measures to avoid chilling, then shrug your shoulders and forget it if you find that you've been uncomfortably cool.

Other people's colds aren't easy to catch. Suppose a stranger sneezes at you in a store. What are your chances of getting a cold?

Actually, almost none at all. Children, who take little care to dodge other people's germs, get colds four times out of five when they are right in the household with a cold victim. But as an adult, you will *escape* four times out of five even if you are in close family contact with a cold. Moreover, most people who sneeze or cough at you in public have already passed the early days when their cold can still be spread, and could not give you germs no matter how hard they tried. Many people sneeze or cough because of conditions which are impossible to spread, like allergy. Your chance of catching a stranger's cold is almost zero, but your chance of worrying yourself into a cold after he's sneezed in your face is considerable indeed, unless you can become convinced that colds rarely spread through such contact.

Cold-fighting morale can really protect you. If you are convinced that nothing is likely to cause colds, you won't suffer psychologically induced ones. You will probably also increase your resistance against whatever cold-causing germs you meet. So whenever you find yourself thinking that what has just happened might cause a cold, repeat to yourself several times: "Nothing that happens to me can give me a cold. Not draughts, not chilling, not even a victim's sneeze! Nothing that happens to me can give me a cold!" As you go about your daily activities, have confidence in your body's powers of resistance. You will still occasionally meet an overwhelming number of cold germs and suffer an infection. But you can throw off the bulk of cold germs without even a sniffle.

ORDINARY SORE THROAT, LARYNGITIS, AND COUGH

More and more mild infections of the upper breathing passages seem to be showing up as sore or scratchy throats instead of ordinary colds. Most victims complain of soreness with slight fever or chilly sensations, headache, and muscular discomfort. After 12 to 24 hours, the trouble spreads both up and down: stuffiness in the back of the nose with some thick mucus usually starts first, then soreness beneath the upper part of the breastbone. A dry, uncomfortable cough is often troublesome, especially at night. The severe complaints usually settle down in about a week, but your throat may feel scratchy and an ordinary day's work may prove unusually fatiguing for two or three weeks.

Most of the measures you would use for a common cold prove helpful here: rest, germ shunning, aspirin, and nose drops and sprays as needed. These further measures give additional relief:

Hot gargles. What is the best solution to use as a mouthwash or gargle? One of my doctor friends settled this question by actually using different preparations, then determining how many germs were left. His surprising conclusion: ordinary salt water works just as well as any antiseptic tested. Reason: all the germs on the surface where antiseptics can reach them wash away promptly anyway. Germs down the sewer do you no more harm alive than dead.

Frequent gargling removes germs. One-half teaspoonful of table salt to a glassful of water is as effective as any gargling solution you can buy. You can add considerably to the soothing effect of gargles by making them quite hot: as hot as you can stand without burning. Hot salt water gargles four times a day help to keep you comfortable and speed your recovery.

Hot irrigations. The rawness of a virus sore throat often extends so far back that gargling just doesn't seem to reach it. In this case, or if you have difficulty gargling effectively, the best home measure is the hot irrigation. Fit the glass tip from an ordinary eyedropper to the end of a household enema apparatus (fountain syringe). Make an irrigating solution by adding four level teaspoonfuls of table salt to two quarts of very warm water, as hot as you can use comfortably without burning (112°F.). Arrange the enema bag 24 inches above the level at which you will irrigate. Lean over a washbasin with your head tipped forward and your mouth open. Squirt the water back into your throat, directing the stream toward the sore area. You won't choke and you need not spit: the water will run back out into the basin. Pause occasionally to breathe. If gagging occurs, direct the stream a bit lower—the problem is usually that the solution has forced the uvula back against the sensitive back wall of your pharynx. Repeat until all the solution is used up.

You can use throat irrigations several times a day for ordinary sore throat. Smoldering throat problems which cause soreness mainly in the morning yield especially well to this measure.

Throat-soothing syrups. An ordinary sore throat soon settles down to the stage of morning rawness and dry, harsh feeling, which yields very well to loosening-type cough syrups. Syrup of cocillana, available at your drugstore in such preparations as Syrup of Cosanyl, works especially well. Cough mixtures containing ipecac and ammonium chloride such as Lilly's Mentholated Expectorant are also effective.

Laryngitis. Virus sore throats sometimes settle in the voice box, causing hoarseness or complete loss of voice and a brassy, tight-feeling cough. In severe cases, or if breathing becomes difficult, you need your doctor's help. The much commoner, mild form of laryngitis often yields to these home measures:

Steam. You can usually get a great deal of relief and definitely speed healing of laryngitis by breathing moist, steamy air for at least half an hour three or four times a day. Make a steam tent on your bed by opening an umbrella, laying it on its side with the top toward the head of the bed, and covering it with a sheet. Put a hot plate on the floor beside the bed, and start a kettle of water boiling on it. Use the core from a roll of paper towels or a rolled piece of heavy wrapping paper held together with several rubber bands to lead the steam up into your tent. Steam gives great help for croup and childhood coughs, many of which are forms of laryngitis. The safety problems of such care make it almost too dangerous to use, though. Youngsters become restless and unreliable when ill. Anything hot in their vicinity becomes a great hazard, either through scalding or through shifting of the sheets or bedclothing into the source of heat. Fortunately, there is a way to eat your cake and have it, too—"cold steamers," which actually work by throwing out a mist of very fine water droplets instead of boiling the water into steam, give just about the same benefits without burn risk. Any drugstore can supply such a unit for about $20—substantial expense, but cheap as insurance against a painful and disabling burn.

Voice rest. A husky voice means that your vocal cords are swollen, red and raw. If any surface part of your body—say your finger—were swollen, red, and raw, you would carefully spare it from any unnecessary use. Why not do the same thing with your voice? Most patients find that if they can absolutely stop talking for two days, carrying a notebook and pencil with which to write notes for essential communications, they usually get well. If this is impossible for you, spare your voice as much as you can.

Warmth. Laryngitis is very sensitive to temperature change. You will get well much more quickly if you stay at home with hoarseness. If you must go out, wear a double muffler or wool scarf around your neck.

Home measures for cough. You can decide which coughs will probably yield quickly to home measures and which need medical attention right away. Your doctor can give worthwhile help if:

1. Your temperature goes over 100 degrees.
2. You get severe headache, aches and pains, and chilly sensations.
3. You spit up bloodstreaked or rusty-looking phlegm.
4. Your appetite is off, so that you are losing weight.
5. The cough is accompanied by pain in the chest, other than a tight feeling under the upper part of the breastbone, by pain on breathing deeply, or by shortness of breath.
6. The cough produces more than two tablespoons of pus-filled or foul-smelling phlegm before breakfast time.
7. The cough fails to respond promptly to home measures.

Tight coughs. When the rawness from a cold or ordinary sore throat spreads down into your windpipe, you get a tight, dry cough. You do not spit up much phlegm or feel it rattling around in your chest as you do with a loose cough. A tearing sensation may clutch at your chest with each paroxysm. Cough may be especially annoying when you first lie down at night, and shortly after any spurt of activity or exertion.

Benzoin and steam. Steam inhalation helps this kind of cough a great deal. A teaspoonful of compound tincture of benzoin makes the steam even more soothing. Benzoin stains the inside of the pan; unless you have an old kettle you want to use for steaming only, it's best to float a shallow tin can or a tray-shaped piece of heavy aluminum foil inside the kettle and put the benzoin inside *that*. Many patients find that steaming for an hour or more four times a day is very worthwhile, although shorter periods also help. If you use this treatment for a child, stay with him or her constantly. Read a story to him to keep down restlessness, and don't turn your back for an instant—the burn hazard from any steam source hot enough to vaporize the benzoin is very real indeed.

Cough syrups. Almost all of the nonprescription cough syrups are cough-loosening agents, and many of them work very well. If you haven't been satisfied with the product you have in your medicine chest now, try taking two teaspoonfuls of syrup of cosillana every three hours. Brown mixture is another excellent and inexpensive cough mixture.

Aspirin. A severe cough often causes enough discomfort to call for relief. Try aspirin or Tylenol first, two tablets if you weigh 150 pounds or less, three if you weigh more.

Many cough syrups include codeine or opium, which reinforce aspirin's pain relief. For children, scale down doses according to the table on page 111.

Patients with tight cough usually ask about chest rubs, greases, counterirritants, and plasters. These may give some relief, but in my experience not enough to make the disturbed rest and discomfort they involve worthwhile. Soaking the feet in very hot water also has some reflex cough-loosening action, but the water must be so hot that patients often burn themselves. For these reasons, I usually advise against these methods.

Loose cough. Mild varieties of loose cough usually are due to mucus and irritants that ooze down from the back of the nasal passages into the throat, windpipe, and bronchial tubes. You can attack this type of cough in several simple ways:

Salt water snuffling. If you keep the material which sweeps back into your throat thin enough, you can swallow it down without a single cough. Simplest technique: mix half a level teaspoonful of table salt in a glass of lukewarm water, pour a tablespoonful or so into the cupped palm of your hand, and snuffle it up into the nose. Repeat until the passages are clear of thick or irritating clots of mucus. Salt water can also be used in an atomizer if one is available.

Better drainage through controlled sleep posture. When you lie on your back, mucus and irritants from your nose run back into your throat and down your windpipe continually. On your side, this action is almost as great. But when you lie face down, your breathing passages drain outward from the bottom of your windpipe to the tip of your nose. Most patients are not comfortable flat on their abdomens when they have a cough, so I usually recommend putting one pillow underneath the right side of the chest and bending the right knee slightly to keep the body about one-quarter rolled toward the left.

Special gravity-aided lung drainage. If you get a deep, loose type cough, you may have a lot of trouble raising all the phlegm that accumulates in your chest. First thing in the morning, and several times throughout the day as moisture begins to accumulate, you should try this program:

> Lie face down across your bed with a footstool or sturdy wooden box at the bedside just beneath your head. Slide forward until only your hips and legs remain on the bed, with your head and chest dangling almost straight downward. Prop your elbows on the stool or box to achieve reasonable comfort, and take several deep breaths or coughs. Remain in this position for about ten minutes, taking a few deep breaths or coughs every two minutes or so. Do not attempt to swallow phlegm that you raise while in this position: keep a basin or a supply of tissues in reach so that you can spit it out.

Cough syrups and remedies. If bursts of coughing disturb your rest or interfere greatly with jobs you simply must do, you need effective cough controlling medicine. Your druggist can sell without prescription several ready-mixed preparations containing completely safe amounts of codeine or other cough-suppressing opium elements such as elixir of terpin hydrate with codeine, or brown mixture with opium. With severe night cough, you may find standard strength cough mixtures do not give enough relief.

Rest. Mild type coughs are still infections, even though they seldom involve germs of a kind your doctor could kill with penicillin. You can definitely build your recuperative powers with rest. Half an hour in bed before supper and ten hours of rest at night is my usual recommendation.

Fluids. The classic advice is to drink lots of juice, water, and pop. Cola beverages, coffee, and tea should not be used beyond the amounts to which you are accustomed, because they contain enough stimulant to cause restlessness or gas cramps when used in large quantity. Ginger ale, fruit flavored pop, and mixtures of fruit juice and ginger ale often sit especially well. Probably the main benefit you get from this program is control of the bowel problems which otherwise often follow upon decreased activity, fever, poor appetite, and constipating medications. I don't advise alcoholic beverages as a means of forcing fluids, since alcohol combines with a great deal of water in the process of burning inside your body (as everyone who has suffered morning-after thirst can tell).

9

How to Control Dragged-out and Recurring Miseries of the Nose, Throat, and Sinuses

Many dragged-out or recurring nose, throat, and sinus miseries cause considerable suffering without quite driving you to your doctor's office. You've more or less learned to live with your smoldering sinus discomfort. Each individual attack of hay fever is half over before you can find time for a doctor visit. So you bear up as best you can.

You'll find that proper home measures make these disorders much easier to bear. You can probably get considerable relief from sore or crusted nose, sinus trouble, and chronic sore throat with simple home measures. Drainage back into your throat with constant tickle or "smoker's cough" may yield entirely to home measures. You may rid yourself entirely of nosebleeds, stuffy nose, hay or rose fever, allergic rhinitis and even asthma with home measures. The rugged Minnesota climate gives us plenty of chance to try different home measures against these ailments. Here are the remedies my patients have found most effective.

NASAL CRUSTING, SORE NOSE, AND NOSEBLEEDS

Some of the most common and most easily corrected nasal miseries stem from the irritating dryness of the air you breathe. The more you heat air, the drier it becomes, which makes the indoor air positively crackle during Minnesota winters. Even in areas with milder weather, nasal crusts or boogies form just inside the nose, causing considerable discomfort and stuffiness. You almost can't help picking at these crusts at times, causing soreness, nosebleeds and infection. Dry air often causes nosebleeds, too: the spot where most nosebleeds start is just inside the nose on the wall between the two nostrils, where the nose lining is stretched thin and easily dried to the cracking point.

121

Nasal crusts. You can probably save yourself a great deal of nagging discomfort by controlling nasal crusts. Moisturizing measures (used for cold prevention, as explained in Chapter 8) may also control crusts. If not, try these techniques:

Nose lining anointment. You can usually prevent all crusting, most nose soreness, and a substantial share of nosebleeds by anointing your nose lining with lanolin or petroleum jelly. Most of my patients use this measure about three times a week during the heating season, and perhaps once a week during warm weather. More frequent self-treatment is perfectly safe if it proves desirable. Here are detailed directions:

> Obtain one ounce of lanolin from your druggist. Dip up a glob slightly larger than a match head with the tip of your right index finger or with a cotton-tipped applicator. Gently press the tip of your nose straight upward with the tip of your left index finger, and apply the lanolin to the front corner of the wall between the nostrils about a quarter-inch up from the opening. As the lanolin melts, it will spread over the entire nose lining layer.
>
> If lanolin is not readily available or if you find its smell objectionable, use *unmedicated* white petroleum jelly. Probably you will need two or three times as many applications of petroleum jelly as of lanolin, but it does just as good a job.
>
> CAUTION: NEITHER LANOLIN NOR PETROLEUM JELLY SHOULD BE USED BELOW AGE TWELVE. Underdeveloped childhood "sweeper" cells cannot handle oily substances, and allow them to trickle down into the lungs, occasionally causing serious disease.

Tap water snuffling. If nasal crusts or dryness already plague you, the temptation to pick or blow at them is almost intolerable. Any measure which softens the crust will let your nose lining's sweeper cells carry them away. If you sniff up a teaspoonful or two of warm tap water from the palm of your hand, you can usually restore nasal comfort without harmful picking or blowing. The high chlorine content makes most tap water slightly more harsh than moisturizing spray, but not harmfully so. The amount of water you can hold on your palm will not fill the cavern of your nose and will not cause gagging or get into your windpipe.

Sore nose. A red, sore swelling of the side of the nose just above the nostril frequently results from pull on the hair roots inside the nose, either by crusts or while clipping protruding nasal hair. If you suffer from this condition, *do not pick or squeeze the sore area.* The veins which carry blood away from this spot lead back through the brain cage in many people. Squeezing or picking can occasionally result in very serious spread of infection along those veins. You can never be sure whether you have the dangerous variety of circulation until too late, so it's best to take no chance of stirring up a brain abscess or other deadly disorder. Instead, use heat to draw out or heal the infection. Apply wet cloths which are as hot as is comfortable without burning (112 degrees), cover with a dry towel to help hold the heat, and change every five minutes or so to keep the temperature right. Each application should last at least half an hour. Every two hours is about the right frequency. If soreness spreads, chills and fever develop, or the tissue around the eye begins to swell, call your doctor.

Nosebleeds. If you have a nosebleed, nine times out of ten it originates in the wall between your nostrils just behind the tip of your nose. To control a nosebleed, try these five steps:

Patience and proper position. By sitting up in a quiet and relaxed position, you cut down the pressure in the nasal blood vessels. This often helps normal processes of repair. Ordinarily, your head should be tipped slightly forward so that the blood runs out of your nose instead of back into your throat. Otherwise, swallowed blood often irritates the stomach, adding nausea and vomiting to your other problems. If you become dizzy or faint in the upright position, you may need to lie down temporarily: if so, lie partly on your face and partly on your side with pillows to support you.

Cold compresses. A cold cloth on the bridge of the nose or forehead sometimes seems to contract the bleeding vessels and help stop them up.

Nasal packs. A half-inch-wide strip of facial tissue or a wisp of cotton helps to give flowing blood a matrix on which to clot. Double the pack over the blunt end of a pencil and insert it gently straight up toward the forehead, about three-quarters of an inch. Touch the pack against the wall between your nostrils, and twist the pencil slightly to disengage it. Withdraw the pencil, leaving the pack in place. Pick up another fold of the pack material two or three inches down and follow the same procedure until the nasal passage is full. No great pressure is required.

Pressure between fingers. If the bleeding continues in spite of the pack, gently press the sides of your nose together between your thumb and forefinger, increasing pressure on the pack. Continue the pressure for at least five minutes by the clock before releasing it to see whether bleeding still continues.

Clothespin pressure. Some patients seem to get better results by using a pincer-type clothespin with a couple of layers of handkerchief for padding, which they leave in place for 10 to 15 minutes.

Removing the pack. If a nasal pack or a pack plus pressure finally stops a nosebleed, you should leave the pack in place for 3 to 12 hours. Otherwise, the bleeding often starts again when you remove the pack. If you have used cotton, you can moisten it with mild salt water (one-half teaspoon to a glassful of water) several times over a five minute period before attempting to remove it. Packing can be replaced if fresh bleeding starts, but should not be left in place for over 24 hours. See your doctor if bleeding continues after that interval.

Follow-up treatment. In most cases, the lanolin program described above prevents further nosebleeds. However, nosebleeds sometimes are due to high blood pressure, disease of the blood, or rheumatic fever, for which medical treatment is very worthwhile. Frequent or severe nosebleeds, or nosebleeds accompanied by other complaints such as headache, joint pains, or fever, certainly deserve your doctor's care.

HOME CARE FOR SINUS MISERIES, STUFFY NOSE, CHRONIC SORE THROAT, AND POSTNASAL DRIP

Sinus blockage or irritation causes pain. Infection which calls for prescription germ killers only occurs in about one-fifth of the cases. Among the patients with complaints severe enough and protracted enough to reach a specialist, a majority have infection. However, a British study based on *all* people with sinus complaints shows that four out of five have germ-free sinuses. My own experience almost exactly duplicates this figure. You can distinguish attacks that require your doctor's prompt attention by these signs:

1. Throbbing pain instead of steady, dull discomfort.
2. Fever.
3. Muscular aches and pains, loss of appetite and weakness.
4. Foul-smelling or opaque white or yellow matter draining back into the throat usually means infection. Translucent or semi-opaque mucus does not necessarily mean infection no matter what its color might be.

Home care when sinus pain strikes. Steady, bursting pain under the cheekbones or just above the eyes usually stems from sinus irritation. If you get such an attack, these measures may help:

Aspirin or Tylenol. Three aspirin or Tylenol tablets help to relieve the average 150 pounder. Adjust the dose up or down if your weight is 35 pounds or more from this standard.

Nose lining shrinkers. Sudafed tablets every eight hours help to shrink the nose lining and open up the sinus cavities. A high percentage of sinus victims also have some allergic component in their miseries, so Contac, Dristan or similar preparations make more sense than they do for plain colds. None of these preparations should be used if you have a blood pressure or heart problem, in which case you should use nose drops in the position described in the last chapter.

Lightbulb baking. Many sinus sufferers find heat quite helpful. One convenient form is lightbulb baking. Place moist pieces of cotton over your eyes. Place 100-watt bulbs in two lamps with metal reflectors, such as goosenecked desk lamps. If you have no lamps with metal reflectors, line the shades of ordinary lamps with aluminum foil. Place the lamps about three feet away from your face, and adjust them closer or farther away as necessary as the bulbs become hot and your face becomes accustomed to the warmth. At least 30 minutes of baking is usually best at a sitting. Treatment can be continued safely for several hours or repeated frequently throughout the day if necessary.

Hot applications. Wet heat sometimes works as well or better than baking. A folded towel dipped in hot water works very well. The water should be as hot as is comfortable without risk of burning (112°). A dry towel or piece of plastic sheeting such as a plastic refrigerator bag helps to cut evaporation and to hold the heat. Dip the towel as often as necessary to keep it hot for 20 to 30 minutes. Always test water temperature with the back of your hand or some part not being treated with heat: otherwise, you may become sufficiently accustomed to the warmth to burn yourself.

Nasal irrigation. To some extent, the thick mucus which has already passed into the nearby nasal cavity blocks drainage. You can remove this material without harmful nose blowing by gentle nasal irrigation. Use nose-drops or spray five to ten minutes before this treatment to open the nasal passages. Mix four teaspoonfuls of table salt with two quarts of warm water in an enema bag. Replace the enema tip with the glass portion of an eyedropper. Insert this part way into one nostril and compress the side of your nose gently with a fingertip to make it fit snugly. Lean your head slightly forward over a basin. Adjust the enema bag so that the water level in it is about 12 inches higher than your nose, and start the flow. Water should run into one nostril and out the other. If flow is sluggish, you may increase the pressure slightly by raising the bag or lowering your head, but *never* allow more than eighteen inches difference in height between the bag and your nose.

Nasal siphonage. If you have frequent or continual sinus misery, an additional refinement may be worthwhile. Attach another eye-dropper tip to a two-foot piece of rubber tubing. Put a little water in your washbasin and immerse this tube in such a way that water displaces all the air from inside. Clamp or pinch off the tube. Prepare for nasal irrigation as described in the last paragraph, fitting the irrigating tip into your right nostril. Fit the siphon tip into your left nostril leaving its free end under water in the basin. Don't let the tubing empty itself. Release both tubes simultaneously. The weight of the water in the downward-flowing siphon tube creates a suction which literally pulls matter out of the sinuses. If the siphonage is interrupted for any reason, refill the siphon tube with water to restore full action. After you have used about half the irrigating solution, clamp or pinch off both tubes again and reverse nostrils to complete the treatment.

How to control continual sinus discomfort, stuffy nose, chronic sore throat, and postnasal drip. If you have continual nose troubles, the chances are that irritation is at fault. If your doctor has never remarked about the wall between your nostrils being far out of line or about other defects of nasal structure, and if the signs of infection which we discussed a few pages back have not been present, these home measures may give considerable improvement:

Stop using nose lining shrinkers, medicated nose drops, sprays, and jellies. Agents which shrink the nasal lining frequently cause rebound congestion, actually causing considerable swelling after a brief interval of relief. Germ-killing medicines and antihistamines often cause later rawness and swelling, too. I have seen patients who continued to suffer from a stuffy nose, postnasal drainage, and sinus pain over long periods—in one case, twelve miserable years—when discontinuing all nasal decongestants, germ killers, and antihistamines brought prompt relief. Long-continued nasal stuffiness often disappears completely or substantially improves if you cease using all such preparations for two weeks. You can make the uncomfortable trial period somewhat more bearable with moisturizing spray and hot applications.

Moisturizing spray. You will probably find that soothing home-made moisturizing spray (formula on page 113) will help you with most smoldering nose and sinus miseries. In addition to its cold-fighting action, this preparation thins thick, mucoid matter which drains back into the throat in almost all forms of smoldering nasal trouble. Moisturizing spray lets you swallow draining material easily instead of having it hang through a dozen swallows or coughs. The thin glycerin film left by moisturizing spray helps to replace the normal moving mucus blanket which has often disappeared after long bouts of nasal trouble and medication. It startlingly helps many patients with a background of stuffiness and sinus misery through the years.

Restrain nose-blowing. Besides its infection-spreading effect, violent nose-blowing irritates the nasal lining and makes it become swollen and sensitive. Sometimes this leads to a vicious circle: more swelling and sensitivity causes stuffiness and annoyance, which makes you blow your nose, which causes still more swelling and sensitivity. Either don't blow, or if you must blow keep both nostrils open and blow gently. Perhaps salt or tap water snuffling will help get rid of secretions, too.

Use a chin binder if necessary. Morning sore throat often results when your mouth drops open during relaxed sleep, so that you breathe through your mouth instead of your nose. Try moisturization and lowered nighttime temperature. If these measures fail, tie a soft cloth around your chin from the top of your head to hold your mouth closed when you are completely relaxed.

Tunnel breathing and protective clothing. Your nasal lining may be quite sensitive to abrupt changes in temperature and humidity. Sometimes sinus membranes engorge themselves when cold air hits the overlying skin. If you are very subject to such difficulties, you need to protect your face and breathing passages from the cold.

Research aimed at helping people survive in the arctic wastes has produced one excellent answer to this problem: tunnel breathing. In the frozen North, this is done through a fur-lined tunnel which projects forward from a heavy hood. When you take a breath inside such a hood, most of the air you get is warm, moist air which you just breathed out into the hood and tunnel. Just enough fresh air enters to keep your body well supplied.

The hardy Minnesota lumbermen learned many years ago to accomplish the same goal with a properly arranged muffler or scarf. By winding a turn over an ordinary peaked cap, then bringing it loosely over the lower half of the face, they made a breathing tunnel that also served as a sheltered peep hole through which to view the snow covered wonders of our wintry world. If you use a scarf in this way, be sure to wind it so that you rebreathe warm air trapped in your peep hole tunnel instead of breathing through the material.

The plastic masks which many surgeons now use in place of the old gauze models have much the same effect. Air comes into your breathing passages only after having passed through a narrow, tortuous path across your warm cheek surfaces. The 3 M Company marketed "cold weather masks" of this type widely for a while, too. Although they didn't go over too well with the general public, some drugstores still have these in stock.

Waxen kernels. Smoldering infection in the throat or sinuses often shows up more through sore and swollen glands down the neck than through direct soreness. This is especially true of children, in whom waxen kernels may stand out like knots beneath the angles of the jaws. Use the same measures with waxen kernels you would apply to chronic sore throats or sinus, as above. These lymph glands are the filters with which your body catches germs as they try to invade your system. Clearing up the germ source gets rid of gland infection more readily than any treatment aimed at the glands themselves, and hot soaks or other measures may make the glands drain through the skin, leaving unsightly scars.

If lymph glands enlarge without clear-cut infection of the nose or throat or if enlargement persists, blood counts and other studies should be done. This means a doctor visit, of course.

Antihistamines. A stuffy nose often stems from allergy to dusts and pollens or from irritation by fumes, dry air, cold air or emotional upset. You can usually get relief from all of these types of congestion with antihistamine tablets or capsules, some of the best of which are now available without a prescription. Most of my stuffy nose patients need about four capsules a day. They usually take their medicine immediately after meals and at bedtime to avoid the slight indigestion which antihistamines sometimes cause when taken on an empty stomach. A few people get a little dopey or slow from antihistamines, so you should always take the first dose when you do not have to drive a car or operate dangerous machinery for a few hours.

Corrective measures against allergy. Smoldering nasal complaints of any sort may have an allergic background. Such origin is especially likely if:

Stuffiness and discharge are worse in the morning when you first get up. Even if sinus pain occurs later in the day, signs of nasal irritation first thing in the morning may mean that the whole problem is due to allergy.

Watery discharge, sneezing, and stuffiness follow tasks involving exposure to household dusts, visits to certain localities, or nearness to certain objects. Anything from Grandma's cat to mold in a moist basement may be responsible.

Complaints clear up during vacation trips or visits away from home, or vanish when you take antihistamines.

If your complaints might be related in any way to allergy, here are nine tried and true home remedies, which my patients have found helpful.

HOME MEASURES AGAINST ALLERGY

Minnesota's fabulous variety of trees and grasses, plus a profusion of weeds on its vast stretches of uncultivated land, make pollen allergy one of its commonest plagues. House dust, animal dander, and molds bother our hearty Swedes as much as other Americans, too. When one of my patients complains of frequent nose colds with no fever or muscular discomfort, I can be almost sure that he really has allergy instead of infection. Continual watery discharge, nasal stuffiness, and sneezing point toward allergic rhinitis, the perennial form of hay fever which allergy sufferers tend to develop either independently or as an aftermath of the pollen allergy season. Asthma and hay fever almost always stem from allergy to breathed-in substances, of course.

Home measures help tremendously in fighting these varieties of allergy-caused misery. As emergency aid when you suffer an attack, *antihistamine capsules or tablets* every four hours often bring relief. *Ephedrine,* either in capsule form or in half-teaspoonful swallowed doses of the standard one per cent nose drop solution, is very helpful for either nasal allergies or asthma unless you have heart disease or high blood pressure. Some patients find that ephedrine makes them very restless, especially if they take it in the evening. A quarter of any commonly prescribed sleeping tablet helps to cancel out this action.

These measures frequently will get you through an occasional mild attack. If your allergies cause frequent or severe trouble, your doctor can offer more effective and convenient remedies.

Long-range relief from asthma, hay fever, and allergic sinus or rhinitis. Home measures to remove or trap allergy-causing substances often bring even severe asthma or nasal allergy under control. Dust, pollen, molds and chemicals aggravate every form of breathing passage allergy. These steps often improve or completely relieve allergic distress:

1. Sponge away dust. As a starter, you should get rid of all the accumulated dust (and the pollen which clings to it) from hidden corners of your living quarters. This is one job which you will probably have to get someone to do for you: you can't usually do it yourself without bringing on a disabling allergic attack. A wet sponge or cloth should be the main dirt-removing weapon, since dust cloths only rearrange the dirt without getting rid of it. All drapes, curtains, hangings, and rugs should go into the wash, to the cleaners, or out in the yard for vacuuming, home dry cleaning, or soap-and-water cleansing. All pictures, framed mirrors, and the like should be taken down, washed or sponged off, and stored away until Operation Dust-Removal is complete. Go over the furniture—top, bottom, outside, and inside—with an oiled or damp cloth. Vacuum each part of each piece of upholstered furniture, and wipe off each coil of every exposed spring. Remove and sponge or vacuum every item from closets, cupboards, and bookshelves. Get all the dust off of walls and ceilings with thorough sponging. Radiators, hot air registers, and heat ducts are terrific dust-catchers, too.

Once the original job is done, you can probably keep ahead of dust accumulation for yourself for another year. You can use a good vacuum cleaner, although you may have to get someone else to empty the bag. Never sweep or dust dry surfaces: if you want to sweep, soak torn bits of paper in ordinary water and scatter them liberally on the surface to be cleaned. Hit all the dust-catching surfaces in one room or area each week, taking the different parts of the house in rotation. If housecleaning makes you distinctly worse, maybe you can trade chores with someone else in the family.

2. Dispose of dust-catchers and holders. Stuffed toys, big rugs in the bedrooms, and lined drapes which need dry cleaning are dust traps. Washable toys, scatter rugs and light, washable curtains or drapes are usually cheaper than medicines to control your allergies. Or as a last resort, you can simply do without.

3. Settle dust and allergens. You can make most dust and pollen settle out of the air before you breathe it. The less air motion inside your house, the better. That means windows closed tight and doors promptly shut both winter and summer, especially in your own bedroom and living quarters. Oil type furniture polish and oil-containing sweeping compound also help to keep down dust by ensnaring it.

4. Filter out dust and allergies. An air conditioner or electrostatic air cleanser removes many allergens. If you get your doctor to recommend such equipment in writing before you purchase it, cost and maintenance expense usually come off your taxable income, too. Filters for each register are well worthwhile if your heat circulates through ducts.

5. Seal dust-blowing cushions and springs. The biggest single group of dust traps in your home is probably cushions, springs, mattresses and pillows. Every time you sit or lie on such equipment, it acts like a bellows blowing clouds of dust and pollen all around you. The very least you should do is fit all pillows and mattresses in your bedroom with plastic allergy covers. A layer of heavy plastic or oilcloth underneath cotton slipcovers and a sheet of light linoleum tacked to the bottom of each piece of overstuffed furniture may save you a lot of misery, too. You can coat rugs with special dust seal compound. If you have the extra money, foam rubber mattresses and pillows are very comfortable for many allergy sufferers.

6. Seal dust and pollens out of your living quarters. You can't clean all dust and pollen out of attics, cellars, and the great outdoors. But you can often seal these spaces off from your living quarters. A roll of masking tape from any paint or hardware store will seal window cracks, attic doors, and other openings quite thoroughly.

7. Check chemicals. Any chemical substance in your house, from nail polish remover to floor wax to fiberglass insulation (which contains formaldehyde), might be aggravating your allergies. Best first step in finding out which ones you need to replace: take one room each week, and either stay out of it or (in case of your bedroom and such) pack away all the dispensable chemicals in it. If you get better during any one week, try re-introducing one chemical substance every three days until you find all the offenders.

8. *No more pets or posies.* A cat or canary gives a lot of comfort, but not enough to make it worth the risk for allergy sufferers. Likewise, dogs, parakeets, and so on. If you must have something alive around the house, try tropical fish.

Cut flowers and house plants also cause many allergic attacks. Best do without them, at least until your allergies have cleared up. Then you can bring in one plant at a time, so long as new complaints do not appear.

9. *Outdoor sports.* If you like to swim, three precautions will help: stick to warm water and warm weather, use natural bodies of water instead of chlorinated pools, and avoid calm, unagitated pools. This last precaution is based on the fact that a concentrated layer of pollens and allergens gathers at the surface of a calm pool during the night, and remains until it is dissipated by either wave action or considerable swimming and splashing.

Golf, rides in the country, and other sports involving the great outdoors have considerable risk for allergic people during their seasons. If you must try such sports, take an antihistamine tablet half an hour beforehand.

COLD SORES AND FEVER BLISTERS

If you have a tendency toward cold sores, you will get painful blisters which break and leave open sores on your lips with every cold or fever, and sometimes in between. These sometimes will be accompanied by gum sores (see p. 138). You may feel a burning pain and oversensitivity of the spot for a few hours before the blister comes out.

A virus which is present on almost everyone's skin causes these sores. Any time your resistance drops, this virus attacks your tissues. There are two ways to help the situation: by increasing resistance and by soothing the sore when it has already appeared.

Extra zinc. Recent studies have shown that cold sores heal much more rapidly and are less likely to recur if you keep your body's zinc level up. You can obtain zinc in tablet form in a nutrition center, or can find several vitamin-mineral capsules (such as Vi Con C) which contain it at your drugstore. About 80 mcg/day should do the trick.

Tincture of benzoin. An old Swedish nurse told me about this treatment. She had been using tincture of benzoin as a skin toughener before applying adhesive tape and happened to include a fever blister in the painted area when one of her patients was being bandaged for facial cuts. The victim got so much relief that she has been painting cold sores with benzoin ever since. After trying her discovery, so have I.

Either ordinary or compound tincture of benzoin is available in any drugstore without a prescription. Just paint the cold sore three times a day and let it dry. One caution: blisters which have cloudy fluid in them and burst to form a crusted sore, especially with a thick, crumbly brownish crust, may be impetigo instead of cold sores. Particularly in children (and especially if there are infants in the household, because impetigo is infectious and the very young get terribly sick with it), you should double check apparent cold sores which meet this description.

10

Quick Relief for Headache and Tooth, Eye, or Ear Trouble

When a city man with headaches comes to our tranquil lake resorts, he usually leaves his head pain behind. As the last boat pushes off for the bass-haunted lily pads, the happy vacationers seldom see Mr. Resort Owner's careworn face.

"There they go," he's saying to himself. "If the stupid fish don't like the plugs they've brought along, chances are I'll go broke next season!"

So headache remedies don't go begging even in the land of Hiawatha. If anything, the wide open spaces call for more home treatment for headache, toothache, earache, and other miseries. Unless there's a doctor vacationing nearby, North Country people have to depend heavily on their medicine chests. Fortunately, home measures generally give quick and lasting relief.

HEADACHE REMEDIES

Headache often accompanies infection, high blood pressure, kidney trouble, and the like, besides plaguing you independently. You should call your physician promptly whenever headache is accompanied by other signs of disease, such as fever, dizzy spells, nausea, impaired vision, loss of wind on one flight of stairs, swelling of the ankles, or pounding of the heart. Use aspirin, cold cloths, and rest in a darkened room for temporary relief until the doctor comes. For most other headaches you can safely stick with home remedies unless the pain becomes severe or recurs frequently.

Children often complain mainly of headache at the onset of any infection from stomach flu to strep throat. A few specific questions, like "Does it hurt when you swallow?" and "What happens when you take a deep breath?" help you to figure out what the underlying cause might be. Always check for stiff neck, which might point to meningitis or nervous system disease. You might want to hold back on aspirin until you are fairly sure whether you are dealing with a mild virus or a more serious problem.

Pain relief might keep any of you from realizing how bad things are. Moreover, making a youngster feel better makes it almost impossible to keep him totally quiet. Since this is often the most important element of cure, your youngster may be better off with enough discomfort to keep him down than with the prolonged and serious consequences of over-activity.

Home remedies for headache. Aspirin or Tylenol is everybody's first thought for headache. Two tablets often do the trick. Another two-tablet dose may help if the pain persists after two hours. Buffered aspirin has no real advantage. Excedrin combines aspirin with an ingredient which has both mood-lifting and blood-vessel shrinking effects, and sometimes proves effective.

You can get considerable help from other home measures for several varieties of head pain.

Headaches from fatigue or tension. Most dull, nagging headaches stem from fatigue or tension. Although the pain feels definitely inside, the actual trouble lies in tense scalp muscles and congested veins. In addition to aspirin, these measures often help:

Rest in a darkened room. Rest in a darkened room often helps you to win prompt relief from headache. Patients usually find that they can rest better with no pillow or with a very small pillow or rolled towel placed under the neck. Use your large pillows under your legs, arranged so that the shins are roughly parallel to the floor, and under the lower portion of each arm.

Hot towels. A hot, wet towel relaxes painful scalp muscles and speeds circulation through congested vessels. Fold a towel until it is six to eight layers thick. Dip it in water which is as hot as you can stand without the risk of burning (112° F.). Wring out extra moisture. Apply to the painful area and cover the wet towel with a dry one to help hold the heat. Dip the towel in hot water every five minutes or so to keep it hot.

Fingertip massage. You can give very effective headache-soothing massage for yourself, although it is still more effective if you can relax completely while someone else strokes your scalp. Start immediately after a hot towel treatment. Use rhythmic strokes with both hands. Sit up with your fingertips pressed gently at the center of your forehead, the fingers limp and the hands parallel to the floor. Brush your fingertips across the forehead, back above the ears to the back of the head. Turn down the neck and follow your jaw line back to the vicinity of the voice box. Repeat rhythmically, with very gentle pressure.

Postural headaches. Although most people picture Minnesotans as rugged outdoorsmen, we have our share of desk workers, too. Secretaries, typists, clerks, and other people whose work involves long periods of sitting erect in almost unchanged posture frequently get dull afternoon headache. These postural headaches stem from the pressure of strained neck muscles on the roots of nerves which lead to the scalp area. Aspirin, heat, and massage give quiet relief, but discomfort comes back almost every working day until you take steps to prevent it.

Postural training is the biggest single preventive step. Straighten out the curve of your neck by stretching the back of your head toward the ceiling and simultaneously pushing your chin back and downward as if you were trying to tuck it under your head. Remind yourself continually of this new way of balancing your head for a few days, and soon it will become automatic.

Another helpful measure is to rearrange your desk so that you can do different jobs in slightly different position, at least some of them with your head supported on one hand. If these measures fail, use the neck stretching sling described in Chapter One.

Caffeine withdrawal headaches. Midmorning headaches which plague you on rushed and hectic days may stem partly from missing your usual cup of coffee. Anacin gives quick relief because it contains caffeine, which aspirin does not. Take two tablets at the onset of pain.

Low blood sugar headaches. Steady, dull headaches, which plague you when you wake up in the morning or at the time when your blood sugar sags two or three hours after a sugar-loaded or starchy meal, usually respond quickly to any sugar-containing food. Some patients complain of considerable dizziness with low blood sugar headaches, and others feel weak or sleepy. All these symptoms clear up in five minutes or less if you take a glass of sweetened orange juice or a couple of soft mints. If you are highly subject to such complaints, carry a package of "lifesavers" or some mints at all times. For quick absorption, chew them up instead of sucking them.

If sugar gives quick relief from headaches, dizzy spells or weakness, you almost certainly have hypoglycemia. Chapter 2 gives a full program for controlling this condition, which will give you considerable extra benefits besides control of the head pain.

Migraine headaches. Although severe migraine certainly calls for a doctor's care, some attacks yield well to home measures. The three main features that help you recognize a migraine attack are preliminary warning sensations, throbbing pain often centered on one side, and frequent nausea or vomiting with attacks. The commonest preliminary warning sensations are shiny spots in front of the eyes, distinctive odors, or crawling skin sensations. The pain may strike quite suddenly or increase gradually over a period of an hour or more. Not quite half of the victims vomit with each attack, but many of the others complain of nausea. Tension kicks off many attacks, so that the soothing tonics you will read about in Chapter 14 often help.

Strong coffee. Migraines or any other type of throbbing headaches usually stem from engorged blood vessels. Strong coffee helps to shrink those vessels. One or two cups of strong coffee usually do enough good through this effect to make up for their jitters-spurring action. In severe attacks with nausea and vomiting, you sometimes can get relief by cooling a cup of strong coffee and taking it very slowly as an enema, retaining it as long as possible.

Ice bags. Ice also helps to shrink engorged blood vessels. Ice bags should be padded with a dry towel or a knitted or flannel bag to prevent ice burns. If you do not have a rubber ice bag, a plastic refrigerator bag works fairly well. Apply the ice for 20 minutes at a time, allowing the skin to rest for at least 10 minutes between applications.

Aspirin or Tylenol. Use aspirin or Tylenol, not A.P.C. or other compounds in conjunction with the coffee cure. Three tablets help dull caffeine jitters and fight pain. If you weigh 150 pounds or more, take four tablets for an initial dose.

Rest. Rest in a darkened room helps migraine and other throbbing headaches considerably. Some of my patients have even found eye shades worthwhile.

Diet. During a migraine headache, most patients do not want any food. Warm broth, moderately chilled (not ice cold) ginger ale, or juice may sit fairly well. Avoid very hot and very cold foods for 24 hours.

Prescription medicines. Besides remedies for migraine itself, you might ask your doctor about anti-nauseants and nerve settlers which make fine supplements to other migraine control measures.

Eyestrain headaches. Eyestrain can cause either throbbing or steady headaches, as well as nausea, dulled concentration, and dizziness. Aspirin and rest usually give quick relief. You can usually avoid further trouble through these measures:

Light your work well, at least one-fifth with indirect or bounced light to avoid harsh shadows.

Turn your workbench or chair away from patches of gloom or glare. Excessive contrast greatly increases eye fatigue. This same principle demands some soft light in the room while you watch TV.

Sit up with your work or reading matter held straight in front of you.

If eyestrain headaches continue, have your eyes examined to see if new glasses would help.

HOME MEASURES FOR TOOTH TROUBLES

You can usually relieve a toothache with home measures, at least until you can get further dental care. You can cut down the number of cavities requiring expensive and uncomfortable care. You can slow or curb the tooth socket and gum disorders which cause more lost teeth than all other dental diseases put together.

How to relieve a toothache. Aspirin or Tylenol and well-padded ice bags give some relief from cavity-caused toothache, which you can spot by recalling recent twinges of pain when eating sweets and by finding a brownish or dead-white crater in the shiny enamel of the painful tooth. These further measures are worthwhile:

Oil of cloves. Mild toothache often responds to warm oil of cloves. Pour a little oil into a teaspoon. Warm it with a match. Dab it onto the cavity area with a toothpick or wooden matchstick.

Zinc oxide-oil poultice. Oil alone will not seal larger cavities. Mix up a thick paste of zinc oxide powder and oil of cloves for these. Press a glob of this mixture into the cavity area with your fingertip, then clean off the excess from the surrounding area with the blunt end of a toothpick.

Abscessed teeth. Probably the main thing to do about abscessed teeth is to recognize them so that you don't suffer along for several extra days. A swollen jaw, throbbing pain and some fever usually mean abscess. You can usually spot abscess without swelling or fever by tapping on each tooth in turn with some small metal object when you get pain. An abscess hurts when you tap on the tooth from which it took its start. You can usually get relief for a few hours until you see your dentist by taking two teaspoonfuls of paregoric and full doses of aspirin. A well-padded ice bag also helps.

Soft teeth. If you have a tendency to form cavities very easily, you can probably save yourself considerable misery and expense with these three measures:

Flouride coating. Although fluoridated water does little or nothing for adults, you can harden your tooth enamel at any age by painting it with fluoride. Your dentist can apply strong solutions to your teeth. A safe home corrective for soft teeth is toothpaste which contains stannous fluoride. Brush throughly enough to work the lather across every surface of every tooth daily for about a one-third reduction in cavities.

Diet. A low sugar diet for six to eight weeks can cut your rate of cavity formation for about two years. You can use sucaryl or other calorie-free sugar substitutes to make this program easier. Avoid between-meals eating, sugar-sweetened beverages and desserts for eight weeks, then count the savings in your dental bills.

After-meal mouth rinse. You can cut the number of acid-forming germs in your mouth very substantially by rinsing out your mouth. Take a mouthful of water at the end of each meal and after each between-meals snack or sweetened beverage. Swish the water around your mouth and between your teeth several times, then swallow it or spit it out. This simple technique removes as much as ninety per cent of the germ-breeding food residues from your mouth, and substantially reduces cavity formation. It is especially worthwhile if you cannot brush your teeth after each meal.

Home measures against periodontitis. You can substantially reduce infection of the gums and tooth sockets, which causes a tremendous number of teeth to be lost, with simple home measures. Periodontitis shows up as soreness or tenderness of the gums, sometimes with bleeding. In some cases, loosening of the teeth and tenderness on chewing are the first warning signs. Even if the disease has reached the stage where teeth are quite loose, however, you can often get them to tighten up again with proper care.

Fingertip massage. You usually have to start fingertip massage gradually, since periodontitis makes your gums tender. Begin with one minute of massage twice a day. Moisten the tip of your index finger and reach back inside your cheek but outside of your teeth. Press your fingertip firmly against the upper gum as high up and as far back as possible. Slide the fingertip down toward the teeth. Relax the pressure and return your finger to a spot above the next tooth or space. Press and slide the fingertip downward again. Continue in this manner all the way around the outside of the upper gum. Follow a similar procedure with the lower gum, massaging firmly with strokes beginning far down on the gum and sliding toward the tooth crests. Open the mouth wide. Use small circular motions to massage the inside surface of the gums. If you have a tendency to gag, pant in and out while working far back in the mouth. After finishing fingertip massage, chew on a moderately heavy rubber band for two minutes or so as you go about your business, being especially careful to chew with all available grinders. Don't spare slightly loose or tender teeth.

Toothbrush massage. After two or three weeks of fingertip massage, you may want to start using toothbrush massage, too. Toothbrush strokes should always start well up on the gum and sweep downward toward the tooth points. Ten strokes in each area with a firm brush stimulates circulation considerably.

Gum sores. If you are subject to gum and mouth sores when you are tired or have an upset stomach, you know just how painful they can be. Ordinary sores with a whitish coating and rim of reddish tissue respond well to home measures. If the whitish portion looks leathery, the edges seem heaped-up, or the sores do not heal inside two weeks, see your doctor.

Silver nitrate. If you treat mouth sores right away, you can often shorten their course considerably with silver nitrate. I usually moisten the tip of a cotton-tipped applicator with 10% silver nitrate solution, which you can get at any drugstore without a prescription, and hold it in gentle contact with the ulcer for 5 or 10 seconds, then get the patient to rinse out his mouth with a little water. If you try this technique, use sparing amounts of the solution and keep it right in the sore, since it may otherwise harm the normal surrounding tissue slightly. Keep the silver nitrate separate from other medicines and in a place that is safe from children, since it is quite poisonous.

Gly-Oxide(R). This patent medicine remedy is available in any drugstore without a prescription and works rather well for canker sores, gum sores, irritation from denture rub and so forth. It is packaged in an applicator-top bottle, which makes it easy to apply directly to the sore. Put it on four times a day, following the package directions.

Salt water mouthwash. Whether you apply silver nitrate or not, you can keep down soreness and secondary infection by washing your mouth out thoroughly with mild salt solution three or four times a day. Half a teaspoonful of table salt to a glass of warm water is very soothing.

Gum boils. A sore spot or area on the gums which is red and swollen may be a gum boil. Sometimes a tooth abscess will also drain this way. Aspirin and an ice bag may give temporary relief, but you almost always need some help from a dentist to clear up these conditions.

WATCH FOR EYE DANGER SIGNALS

You can care for many eye troubles for yourself with well-chosen home measures, but you should first check for evidence of possibly serious conditions before you try any treatment on inflamed or painful eyes. See your doctor promptly if any of these signs show up:

Pain in the eyes, over the eyes, or in the back of the head. Abrupt increase in pressure within the eye may cause intense pain. Smoldering cases of glaucoma cause less violent discomfort, which may come and go. Pain starts or becomes worse when the pupils grow larger: in darkness or during an emotional upheaval.

Halos around lights. A rainbow band around street lamps on a clear night may be due to early glaucoma. If you see your doctor promptly, you'll probably be cured without operation and with no loss of vision.

Abrupt worsening of vision. After age 40, your eyes should not change size and shape enough to make you need new glasses more than every two to five years. If either your distant or your close vision becomes notably more blurred within a six-month period, check with your eye doctor to see whether glaucoma or eye changes due to diabetes, high blood pressure, or hardening of the arteries might be responsible. Your doctor can give you help with all of these problems.

Eyes that thrive in gloom. If you see much better in a dimly lit room or with dark glasses, the reason may be a cataract. Cataracts are cloudy spots in one of your eye's light-gathering parts. They often start in the center of the pupil. When you are in a brightly lit room, your pupil becomes smaller so that the still-clear parts of your eye's light-gathering apparatus are blanked out. Result: dim vision in well-lit rooms, better vision in gloom.

A magenta band. If infection or injury involves the clear window into the eye or the deeper tissues, a dusky magenta band about a quarter of an inch wide shows up on the white of the eye around the iris. Sometimes you have to look very closely to distinguish this from the overlay of pinkish inflammation involving the whole white of the eye, which comes with any condition involving rubbing or congestion. If you can't be sure, let your doctor put in some drops which blank out this confusing overlay.

HOME CARE FOR EYE TROUBLES

How to remove a cinder from your eye. When something gets into your eye, tears form immediately to help wash it out. You can aid this normal body mechanism, use other washing techniques, or get someone to remove the cinder for you by flipping the lid. Here are detailed directions:

Aiding your tears. As soon as something flies into your eye, you should close the lid gently and place your fingertip on the lashes. Press straight down along the front of your cheek bone, so that the upper and lower lids both pull slightly away from the eyeball and make a pocket in front of the eye. Let this reservoir fill with tears. Without moving your finger, snap the upper lid open. Then move your finger and allow the lower lid to recoil. Usually the cinder will float out with the accumulated tears.

Eyewashes. Stir one teaspoonful of boric acid powder into a glass of warm water. If any powder is left, let it settle to the bottom and be careful not to get it into your eye. Fill an eyedropper with the overlying clear fluid. Lean your head back and hold both lids of the affected eye as far open as possible with your thumb and forefinger. Squirt the solution into the eye. Repeat three or four times if necessary.

Lid flipping. If milder measures fail, you need to get help from a friend or member of your family. Have your helper carefully search for the cinder on your eyeball by pulling the lower lid down. If he is unable to locate it, the cinder is probably inside your upper lid. Look down without closing your eye. Have your helper grasp your upper eyelashes between his thumb and forefinger. He can then press the side of a pencil point or a small key straight into the lid about an eighth of an inch above the lid margin. The cartilage pad inside the lid, which is perhaps a half inch wide, will flip down over the pupil. By stretching the skin of the lid slightly from the sides, your helper can keep the lid cartilage from flipping back into place while he dabs at the cinder with the corner of a clean handkerchief. If the lid fails to flip back as soon as he lets go, you can replace it easily by opening the eye extra wide with your thumb and forefinger.

Tired eyes, TV eyes. If you are subject to eye fatigue, rest breaks may help. At the end of the first paragraph of every fourth page while you are reading, stop for a moment, let your head nod, and close your eyes. You will feel the tiredness flow out of them over a period of a few seconds, after which you can start reading again. Use commercials for eye rest instead of household chores or conversation when you are watching TV. You will find that a few seconds' break gives your eyes a fresh start.

Salt water rinsing. If you suffer from eye fatigue in spite of brief rest breaks, try salt water rinsing. Let some water stand overnight in an open basin so that all the chlorine escapes. Add a level teaspoonful of table salt to a pint of water. Be sure all the crystals are thoroughly dissolved, and that there is no dirt in the solution. Keep it in a stoppered bottle in a fairly cool place. When your eyes become very fatigued, put some of the moderately cool solution in an eye cup and wash your eyes with it, each for a few moments.

Bloodshot or burning eyes, including pink-eye. Burning, irritated, bloodshot eyes call for mildly astringent drops or ointment. The form of mild eye inflammation which spreads from person to person also yields to these medications. Here is the formula I usually recommend, which druggists in some states can supply without a prescription:

> Zinc sulfate ¼ per cent.
> Saturated solution of boric acid 1 oz.

Put two drops in each eye three or four times a day. Like many potent eye drops, this burns when you first put it in. Don't be alarmed: the burning will quickly subside.

Some patients prefer to use an eye ointment instead of drops. Zinc sulfate ½ per cent works quite well. If you try to put in an eye ointment for yourself, lie down and hold the lids apart. Brace the tube-squeezing thumb against the bridge of your nose. Squirt an amount of ointment equivalent to a small green pea in the inner corner of your eye. In a few seconds, it will melt and spread across the eye. Then you can release the lids and wipe off the surplus ointment with a clean handkerchief.

Sties. Hot cloths help to bring sties to a head. Mild antiseptic ointment helps to keep the germs from one sty from ultimately causing another.

Hot cloths. Fold an ordinary washcloth to four layers' thickness. Dip in water which is as hot as is comfortable (112 degrees) and wring partially dry. Apply to eye, and cover with a dry towel to help hold the heat. Change as often as necessary to keep the cloth hot for twenty minutes.

Antiseptic ointment. If you can get an antiseptic eye ointment like Bacitracin or Furacin without a prescription in your state, it usually helps. Otherwise, old-fashioned yellow oxide of mercury does fairly well. Apply in the inner corner of the eye three times a day. Let it melt and spread across before releasing the lids. If sties occur frequently or fail to yield to these measures, best check with your eye doctor.

HOW TO MANAGE COMMON EAR PROBLEMS FOR YOURSELF

You can probably control some forms of earache and infection, most accumulation of wax, and the commonest varieties of itching, irritated ear canals without a doctor's help. You should suspect disease for which a doctor's prompt care is probably worthwhile when these signs are present:

1. Running ears.
2. Persistent ringing in the ears.
3. Earache accompanied by fever or hearing loss.

Otherwise, home measures are usually worth a try.

The chewing gum cure. An earache often comes from stopped-up air passages. The tube through which air moves into the middle ear space starts near your adenoids. A cold can puff up these tissues until they block off this air tube. Some of the air inside the ear cavity then soaks into your system, leaving a vacuum which sucks back on the drum, stretching it painfully.

Some of your muscles attach to your ear's inner air tube, and certain chewing motions tend to pull the tube open or milk air bubbles through it. That is the basis for the chewing gum cure's effectiveness. An ordinary stick of gum won't do the trick because the movements required have to be quite wide. An adult should chew three pieces of bubble gum (a child should chew two) for an hour or so at a time two or three times a day. If a stopped air tube is causing the trouble, the ear will usually either "pop" or "crackle" as air comes into it.

This cure is also very effective for the feeling of fullness and discomfort after an airplane ride or a trip over the mountains. Even when you don't have a cold, rapid changes in altitude can create a pressure problem which collapses the ear's pressure equalization tube. Chewing a big wad of gum often opens things up.

Even without fever or throbbing, earache can be due to infection, especially if nose-blowing and sneezing have driven germs up into the ear cavity. Don't stick with the chewing gum cure too long under these circumstances, and check frequently for fever or hearing loss which point toward conditions for which a physician's care should give prompt help.

Home remedies for simple earache. For earaches which come on after wind exposure or other irritation, try these measures:

Ear drops. Olive oil, sweet oil, or dehydrated glycerin gives considerable relief when used as ear drops. Warm a dropperful in a dry spoon, using a match or candle. Test on the back of your hand. Lie on your side with the bad ear up and flood the ear canal with the warm drops. Apply a well padded hot water bottle over the ear to help hold the warmth.

Pain-easing medicines. You probably should stick to aspirin alone if you do not plan to see a doctor right away, so that if the pain persists or grows worse you will be aware that all is not going well.

How to keep ear wax from piling up. You can keep ear wax from accumulating in your ear canal by applying home measures. You can put wax softening solutions into the ear canal with perfect safety (unless your doctor has told you to keep all fluid out of your ears because of a perforated eardrum). Once the wax is soft, the slight back and forth motion of the ear canal that occurs with chewing will usually milk it out of your ears.

Homemade wax-softening solution. You can make and use your own wax-softening solution. Mix three drops of any modern liquid dishwashing detergent with one teaspoonful of warm water. Lie on your left side. Put about half of the solution into your right ear. Let it soak in for about one minute. Turn on your right side, holding a handkerchief over the ear opening to soak up excess solution as it runs out. Put the rest of the solution into the left ear, and let it soak in for one minute. Repeat the whole procedure three times a day for three successive days whenever wax begins to accumulate. If the wax has not worked out after three days, a gentle stream of warm water from an all-rubber ear syringe will often wash it free.

Glycerine. Glycerine softens ear wax quite effectively, if allowed to soak in for five minutes two or three times a day. At the end of this period, direct the stream from your shower into the ear to aid removal of any softened wax (unless you have a perforated drum and have been told to keep water out of the ear).

Wax removing devices. I have developed a special device for removing wax plugs from the ears, which is just going into the clinical trial phase as I am writing this section. The first form to be produced will be sold only to doctors, but perhaps by the time you read this book the device will be available in drugstores.

Boils in the ear canals. If you get severe throbbing or steady pain in the ears without hearing loss or fever, your problem is sometimes a boil in the ear canal. The skin is tied to the underlying cartilage so tightly that very little swelling can occur, yet the pressure of infection causes considerable pain. Main tip-off: ear canal infections hurt when you move the outer ear up and down, while inner ear infections do not.

Ichthyol wick. Old fashioned ichthyol ointment helps considerably for ear boils. The easiest way to keep it in contact with the sore is with a thin gauze wick. Cut an 8″ length of one-inch roller gauze bandage lengthwise in half and work it around in a bit of ichthyol ointment until it is thoroughly impregnated. Double one end of it over a cotton tipped applicator and insert half an inch into the ear canal. Hold the wick in place with the blunt end of a toothpick while you withdraw the applicator. Double another fold of wick in front of the ear opening and push it back into the ear with the applicator. Continue until the ear canal is snugly packed with wick.

A product called Cresatin is probably better than ichthyol, but at the moment most druggists can only sell it on prescription.

Itching or discomfort in the ear canals. Smoldering fungus or bacterial infection of the ear canals commonly causes considerable itching and discomfort. If this condition is severe, you should probably get medical help with it. For mild cases, try this technique:

Burow's wick. Gently work a piece of absorbent cotton back into the ear canal. Get an ounce or more of Burow's solution 1:1000 from your druggist. Keep the wick wet with the solution all through the day and night. Change wicks daily, allowing the ear canal to dry out for an hour or so.

Castellani's paint. If Burow's solution fails, you might try Castellani's paint in exactly the same way. This material stains clothing, linens and everything in sight. Best keep a puff of clean dry cotton tucked in the ear on top of the saturated wick to keep down the mess.

11

How to Fight the Special Ailments of Advancing Years

No matter what your age may be, you'll find the information in this chapter useful. It's particularly helpful to people over sixty.

For many years the Minneapolis Transit Company has had a program of free rides or sharply reduced fares for people who have reached a certain age. So our village elders aren't chained to the TV—they can get to recreation halls or free downtown concerts or special events or volunteer work. The Nicollet Mall, which stretches from the Library at one end to the Auditorium at the other, teems with active, interested older people. Many of my patients in their sixties, and seventies and even eighties could write a diary that would make a teenager jealous with its variety and liveliness.

Perhaps that's why Minnesotans have such a deep interest in the special afflictions of the advancing years. Our "sixty plus" people aren't stashed off in nursing homes or residences—they're actively involved in everything that goes on. When one of them has trouble sleeping or suffers periods of dizziness or confusion or breaks a hip from a fall that shouldn't have caused a serious injury, we all know it. Every doctor in town sees lively women with age-induced irritation of the female organs and active men with digestive misery from decreased muscle tone in the diaphram—these things aren't confined to isolated people in far-off institutions. And the special problems of slowing circulation and difficulty with body temperature regulation come into our conversation virtually every day.

Those are the things this chapter discusses, along with the very effective home measures our long-lived Swedes and Germans have devised to keep them in check.

HOW TO KEEP YOUR MEMORY FROM PLAYING TRICKS

Some years ago, I had the privilege of caring for a man in his upper eighties who had actually fought in the Civil War. He painted the most fascinating word-pictures of events and characters, complete with every minute detail. Seven decades had passed, but he still knows the colors of every regiment, the officers in command, the dates of marches and skir-mishes, and an almost day by day roster of the sick, wounded and dead.

That same man would have had much less vivid recollection two or three decades earlier. Some forms of memory actually *improve* with the passing years: your brain does not pile new signals on top of the old, and it lets your recollection of your younger days work closer and closer to the surface. And instant recall remains unchanged with the passing years—you can generally look up a telephone number at eighty and remember it while you dial as well as you could at fifty. Memory problems with advancing years almost always involve recent events—not immediate and not ancient—and generally "trade off" with improved memory for long-past events.

The question of whether or not you have a memory problem can be difficult to answer. Everyone, at every age, occasionally forgets. An important anniversary catches you unaware, a bill gets mislaid, you go to the grocery store without your list and come back missing two or three crucial items. If these things happen frequently, you might find it worth-while to set up memory-sparing systems and routines. Keep all the bills in one spot and pay them on the first and the fifteenth. Post a grocery list on the kitchen wall, and go shopping every Wednesday and Saturday with list in hand. Get a calendar with lots of space for notes, and jot down future special days, plans and engagements. Organization and routine take a lot of strain off your memory, and help free your faculties for other use. That's just common sense, not bowing to an affliction.

Dehydration Lapses. More serious lapses actually fall into two groups, each of which can be controlled in many cases by proper measures. *Dehydration lapses* are probably the most common, often resulting in periods of confusion or in substantial upset in your way of life. The tricky part about these lapses is that your mind fills in the gaps with reasonable events. You distinctly remember paying that bill or eating eggs and bacon for breakfast or turning right at Sixth Street, but the action you remember didn't happen when you think it did. So you get into hassles with the merchants or the bank, or you neglect your body's nutrition, or you get confused about where you actually are.

The basic problem which causes this particular kind of lapse is in your circulation, not your brain. As arteries change with the passing years, they become less capable of contracting and expanding. The mechanisms which have formerly worked to detour extra blood through your brain with each lowering of the total volume of your bloodstream fluid no longer operate as well. So anything which cuts your circulatory volume starves certain portions of your brain and makes your memory fail. Probably the commonest cause of drop in circulatory volume is abrupt change in external air pressure, which draws fluid into the tissues from the smallest blood vessels. That's why these lapses often occur on air flights or motor trips through the mountains, and often vary with the "high" and "low" barometric pressure of passing weather systems. In some cases, the problem is aggravated by a vicious circle—you seem to recall having had your breakfast orange juice and coffee, so you don't eat or drink "again" when you never had those things in the first place, and further dehydration makes similar confusion about midmorning coffee and lunch.

The cure for dehydration lapses is as simple as it can be: water, fruit juice, lemonade or noncola types of pop. Six or eight glasses of these fluids a day will often do wonders for memory lapses or confusion. Don't use caffeine-containing drinks like coffee and cola-containing pops for this purpose, because the caffeine increases loss of fluid through your urine and may actually make the problem worse. Be especially careful to "soak yourself up" before trips (when you might be tempted to limit fluid so that you won't have to go to the bathroom as often) and when the weather map shows an approaching "low."

This simple remedy often works wonders. Oliver M., for instance, became totally confused when he was sent to a nursing home for convalescence after he broke his hip. He didn't recognize his son or his wife, he didn't know how he got to the institution, and he was terrified at having "lost his touch." When his son and daughter-in-law spent a few hours at his bedside offering him juices and ice water every 15 minutes or so, he became clear as a bell. Once he understood the problem, he was able to handle it for himself, and in a few days was able to go home.

More serious varieties of memory lapse. Although dehydration lapses are much more common than the more serious varieties, you need to be alert for the latter, which require a doctor's help. Brief periods of memory loss which begin almost instantaneously and end fairly abruptly in two to five minutes often come from seizure activity. Prescription medicines like Dilantin often control this type of memory loss completely and with no side effects, making a thorough medical checkup worthwhile. Brief lapses associated with other symptoms of nervous system malfunction such as weakness or paralysis of any part, loss of vision in one area (as to the right), dizziness or incoordination, sometimes stem from a constriction in the main arteries to the brain such as the carotid (located in your neck). Such spells are warning signs of possible impending stroke, but both the spells and the stroke can be warded off by proper care. Modern medical equipment lets doctors actually see the walls of these arteries without X-ray or injections (using sound waves to bounce off the artery walls and analyzing the echoes). If the carotid arteries are at fault, the treatment is sometimes as simple as two aspirin tablets in the morning and again at night, with weight loss if indicated. In more serious cases a simple operation restores flow and solves the problem.

HOW TO COMBAT VAGINITIS, BRITTLE BONES AND OTHER DIFFICULTIES FROM HORMONE LACK

At sixty plus your body has adjusted to the lack of sex hormones and you no longer get menopausal symptoms like hot flashes. But many women and a few men still suffer harmful effects from lack of sex hormones.

Louise Stein's case illustrates the most common complaints.

"I itch just fiercely down below," she told me. "And it's gotten where I'm almost ashamed to go out. I can't sit still, I can't leave myself alone, and I'm afraid all my friends will think I've gone crazy or something."

Louise was a sprightly seventy, slightly bowed in the back but alert and active. Examination showed that the lining of the vagina had become abnormally thin and smooth, with profuse watery discharge. This form of vaginitis commonly stems from hormone lack, so I suggested a vaginal cream containing sex hormones. A few days later, Louise seemed virtually well. Then came time to discuss the next step.

"There are arguments both ways," I told her, "but in your particular case I think there's definite reason to take a tablet of female sex hormones every day."

"Just to keep clear of this itch?" she asked.

"Partly. Estrogens in any form will keep your vaginitis under control, and most people find pills a little handier after the first symptoms are under control."

"But I'm afraid of those hormone pills. Don't they sometimes cause cancer?"

"Perhaps. If you compare figures on a thousand women who are taking hormones with those on a thousand who are not, you'll probably find one more with cancer of the breast or uterus over a period of years. But you'll also find several *less* with heart attacks and only a fraction as many with broken bones. Nobody wants to get an unnecessary cancer, but nobody wants to get an unnecessary coronary or hip fracture, either. When your body shows signs of hormone lack, like your vaginitis and your bowed upper back (which shows weakened bones), the benefits of hormones outweigh the risks. You'll live longer and stay healthier *with* hormones than *without*."

"But why can't I just keep using the cream?"

"You can, if you prefer. Actually the hormones soak into your system from your vagina or even from your skin, so you'll get the same benefits either way. But you'll have the same risks, too."

"You mean the cream can cause cancer, too?"

"Vaginal creams, skin creams—anything with sex hormones in it keeps the uterus and breast tissue more active and makes it slightly more cancer-prone. But considering your total health, the hormones do more good than harm."

Louise finally decided to try hormones in tablet form, and has taken a small dose every day for several years now. She hasn't had any more trouble with vaginitis, and she hasn't had either a coronary or a broken bone. No one can tell exactly how much the hormones do for her, but I'm satisfied in my own mind that she's better off with them than without them.

HOW TO MANAGE COLD FEET AND CHILLINESS

Minnesota winters have a beauty all their own. On a clear cold morning, the air literally sparkles with particles of frost. Wisps of drifting snow chase each other across every open space like dancing spirits. Our hearty Scandinavians delight in winter landscapes and feel invigorated by the brisk air—until their circulation begins to slow, and winter becomes the season of cold-numbed fingers and draughts. When blood pumps more slowly, keeping warm becomes a problem. And sometimes, it seems as if even solid walls don't hold out all the chill. When the mercury dips to twenty or thirty below, most over-sixty folk need to muster a few special tricks and techniques to keep comfortable either indoors or out.

How to warm hands or feet that have become unduly cold. Sluggish circulation makes you more likely to suffer from coldness of the hands and feet. It also makes the "common sense" way of warming up cold body parts downright dangerous. Heat applied directly to the cold part increases its oxygen need without restoring the circulation first. I have seen patients in whom this increased demand tipped the balance to cause actual gangrene and loss of tissue. More commonly, chilblains develop in the warming part, causing intense aching pain for fifteen minutes to half an hour.

You can avoid these difficulties by a simple home method of warming cold extremities. Just apply hot compresses to the cold extremity *well above* the chilled portion. If your hands are cold, put a hot compress around your upper arm. If your feet are cold, apply a hot compress or heating pad to your thighs. Heat applied in this way helps in two ways: since the same nerves and blood vessels are involved, heat on the thigh or upper arm sets off natural reflexes which open up the blood vessels leading through the cold part just as effectively as heat applied to the part itself. And blood coursing toward the chilled part is actually warmed somewhat in transit. These effects increase the flow of warm blood through the affected part *without increasing its oxygen need* and therefore restore comfort much more quickly and safely than direct heat.

How to combat sluggish circulation. Take outdoor activities first. The three key matters are:

> A snugly warm torso.
> Plenty of liquids.
> Activities in the outdoor air.

1. A snugly warm torso. Sven Anderson shook his white mane and said: "I hate to leave Minnesota in the wintertime. I've always loved the bright, crisp days—used to save the outdoor jobs on the farm for January just so I'd be out in it. But now my hands and feet get so cold you wouldn't believe it. And nothing seems to help—down mittens, foot packs, even three pairs of wool socks."

"How about a down vest and a parka?" I asked. "Ever try those?"

"It's my hands and feet that get cold, not my belly."

"That's where you feel it, anyway. Your body has special little shunts in the circulation of your hands and feet to detour blood directly from the arteries to the veins. Those shunts open when your system is trying to save body heat, so that the warm blood won't spread out over all the extra surface of your fingers and toes. This means that when your body is trying to save heat, very little blood goes out to warm your hands and feet, so they get dangerously and uncomfortably cold. The trick is to keep your body from sending those heat-saver signals. If the main parts of your body stay at higher-than-normal temperature, warm blood will always flow all the way through to the tips of your fingers and the ends of your toes. You'll keep your hands much warmer with a heavy sweater and a down jacket than you will with extra pairs of mittens, and the same holds for your feet."

My advice must have worked for Sven. The next time I saw him, he had cancelled his Arizona midwinter vacation and bought a new pair of cross-country skis instead.

2. Plenty of liquids. One of my patients always refers to coffee as "Swedish gasoline." Watching the outdoor workers in the area dip into their thermoses, I can understand the phrase. But it isn't entirely the stimulant in coffee or even the fact that it is piping hot that makes it helpful in combatting cold: it's the simple fact that it is readily soaked-in liquid. Particularly as the passing years slow your circulation, you need a plentiful supply of fluid in your system to "keep the juices flowing."

Actually, coffee isn't the best choice for this mission. As I already mentioned, the caffeine in coffee increases the amount of urine you pass, so that it gives only a temporary boost in circulatory volume, then causes a rebound decrease. Hot bouillon or broth makes the best "winter circulation booster," with plain water, Seven Up, ginger ale or root beer as "also rans." The liquid doesn't have to be hot to do the circulation-boosting job, and even melted snow (in the good, clean wilderness) is better than nothing. Particularly as your years multiply, you'll find that flooding your system with extra fluid before you go out in the cold helps you to remain comfortable in the colder weather.

3. Activities in the outdoor air. When I moved to Minnesota twenty-some years ago, the old-timers absolutely amazed me. People went out in their shirtsleeves on sunny forty degree days and complained about the heat whenever the mercury hit eighty. Now I understand that both these phenomenon stem from the process of acclimation—that the body changes its circulation and heat production to suit the circumstances in which you live. In recent years, my family and I have been swimming when the leaves were falling off the trees and playing tennis in shorts when the snow hasn't melted in the shade, and turning on the air conditioner when a Texan might be turning on the heat. All because of body processes we don't feel and can't measure or control.

You can't deliberately turn on the marvelous process of acclimation and make your body suit itself better to the climate in which you live. But you *can* and probably *should* get into the kinds of activities which make this process occur automatically.

So far as cold is concerned, that means doing something active enough to generate copious body heat while your face and air passages are exposed to the cold. In recent years, I have gone in heavily for cross-country skiing and platform tennis (played outdoors even at 10 below), and I've felt a great deal warmer when outdoors than I did when my main winter sports were performed indoors. Both from my own experience and that of many patients, I'm convinced that undue chilliness and discomfort when exposed to the cold is a vicious circle. If you feel uncomfortable outdoors in the winter, you avoid outdoor activities like the plague. Then your body never adjusts, you continue to feel uncomfortable, and around and around the circle goes. Bundle up, take a brisk walk or do an outdoor task at least once a week as the weather changes from warm to cold. You'll be amazed at how much better you tolerate cold if you get in a few minutes of vigorous activity in it at frequent intervals.

How to combat chilliness and consciousness of indoor draughts.

Although the measures discussed above for surviving outdoor exposure in the wintertime also help you to keep comfortable indoors, heated air introduces one new factor of enormous importance: humidity.

An amazing percentage of the heat loss from your body occurs through evaporation. You've probably become acutely aware of this if you've ever been called to the telephone while you're still dripping wet from a bath or shower. The bathroom air was reasonably moist, but as soon as you hit the dry air in the rest of the house, every wet surface on your body felt freezing cold.

And the air in the rest of the house is usually very dry. When the outdoor air becomes cold, the moisture condenses or freezes out of it. That's the source of the dew or frost you see outdoors in the morning—air holds less and less moisture when it gets colder and colder. So on a really cold morning or day, practically all the moisture has been wrung out of the outdoor air. When that air penetrates into your house and you heat it without adding moisture, you make it exceedingly dry. Actually, you double the air's capacity for moisture (and thus its drying power to your skin and tissues) every 5 degrees. So if air has 50 percent humidity at 0, it will have 25 percent at 5 degrees, 12.5 percent at 10 degrees, 6.25 percent at 15 degrees and so forth.

So you often feel chilly at 70 degrees indoors when the outdoor temperature is 0, even though you would be perfectly comfortable at 70 degrees if the outdoor temperature were reasonably warm. The extreme dryness of the air increases tissue heat loss and makes you chilly, often right up to the temperature at which you feel uncomfortably warm. And as the years pass your circulation becomes less and less capable of adjusting to this situation, and dry heated air becomes progressively more uncomfortable.

The best answer to this problem is humidification. If you can get enough extra moisture in the air to keep the relative humidity above 25 percent, you will feel much more comfortable, and you will also need a lot less expensive heat. An automatic humidifier on the furnace is ideal, but the circumstances may make that solution impossible. If so, a room humidifier, shallow pans of water on the radiators or in the heat ducts, leaving the hot water in your tub with the door open for an hour or so after you bathe, and drying clothes indoors in the basement may all help. As a last resort, try something that seems downright crazy: push that thermostat *down* 5 or 10 degrees. I have several patients who could never get comfortable when the house was heated to 80 degrees no matter what kind of clothing they put on, but they feel perfectly fine with an extra sweater or two in a house heated to 60. The lower temperature makes a 16-fold difference in humidity, and for many people the difference in tissue cooling through evaporation is more important than the difference in tissue warmth from surrounding air.

HOW TO COMBAT SPECIAL
DIGESTIVE MISERIES OF SIXTY-PLUS

"There's no way I should be getting an ulcer," John Wheeler told me. "It's five years since I retired, and I haven't got a worry in the world. Amanda's a lovely woman to live with, my youngsters are all on their own and doing fine. What in the world would give me a pain in the gut?"

"Lots of things besides ulcers. Tell me about it?"

"Almost every night I wake up with heartburn. It aches like hell right in the pit of my stomach. I get up and take a glass of milk, and that soothes it for a while. Then it's more of the same an hour or two after I lie down."

"Sounds like a hiatus hernia. That's a weakness in the diaphragm where your esophagus goes through, so that part of your stomach slides up into your chest cavity."

"You mean its something wrong with the way I'm put together?"

"That's right. The gap in the muscle of the diaphragm probably has been with you for years, but it's quite common to start having problems in your sixties or seventies, or sometimes even later—Pope John had a hiatus hernia, and he didn't have any trouble with it until he was almost eighty."

"Why's that?"

"Probably because the tissues get a little more relaxed and things aren't held as firmly in place. Anyway, there are four things we can do about it. First, you ought to have a set of X-rays. Even though your complaints sound perfectly typical, anybody who has digestive complaints that drag on for any length of time ought to make sure of exactly what's there—it's better to dot the i's and cross the t's than to miss a tumor in the curable stage or treat you for the wrong condition. Second, you should get some blocks about 4 inches high and put them under the head of the bed. Even a little bit of downhill slant helps keep your stomach where it belongs, and four inches is usually about as much as you can take without winding up scrunched down at the bottom of the bed after you've rolled around once or twice. Third, you should take off some weight. Some of the fat deposits in your body are located inside the abdominal cavity, and even a few pounds extra in that particular location pushes your stomach up where it doesn't belong. Last, you can take some antacid like Mylanta after supper and at bedtime to try to soothe the part of your stomach that's rubbed itself raw going in and out through the narrow hiatal defect."

"Sounds like a pretty full program. How long will it take me to get relief?"

"You'll feel somewhat better with the antacids and the bed blocks, but you won't be fully relieved until you lose the weight. If that doesn't do the trick, there's always surgery—sounds like a tough place to get at, but by making the incision between two ribs where it's naturally splinted you can have the hernia repaired with a lot less discomfort and disability than you would expect. I'd say the operation is on a par with getting your appendix out—bad enough to avoid if you can, but easy enough that you shouldn't suffer on month after month to avoid it."

Actually, John Wheeler didn't need an operation. In two weeks his condition had improved enough that he could sleep normally, and in a month he was able to quit antacids entirely. He still sleeps with the head of the bed raised (there's also a wedge-shaped pad available to raise one person's head in a double bed, but John's wife didn't object to the plain blocks). And he's stayed about ten pounds lighter, which I think is the most important thing. If you have symptoms suggesting a hiatus hernia, or if one was found on X-rays in former years and you think you might be having a little trouble with it, try these measures. They usually work very well, and often save later need for an operation.

HOW TO CARE FOR THICKENED NAILS

Your toenails often become a source of considerable minor misery in your later years. Dorothy Peterson, for instance, complained that her nails had become so thick and heavy that they rubbed painfully against the tops of her shoes.

"And I just about can't cut them myself," she told me. "They sort of crack and splinter instead of cutting clean. And I just can't get through them with manicure scissors—I've sprung two pairs trying."

Dorothy's nails were about an eighth of an inch thick with heavy lengthwise ridges. They curved downward a bit at the ends of her toes, but not enough to dig into the flesh (as happens to a few unlucky souls). She had avoided the ingrown toenail hazard, which sometimes afflicts people with heavy brittle nails. The way heavy nails crack and splinter when you try to cut them makes it hard to wind up with a straight nail end.

"I'd suggest two things," I told Dorothy. "First, get a pair of straight clippers. You can find them at any drugstore for under $2. They work just like inexpensive fingernail clippers, with the lever that folds up on the top and the spring steel bodies and blades. Fingernail clippers always have a curved edge, though, and toenail clippers should be straight."

"I've seen some of those, but they didn't look big enough to go all the way across my nails."

"They aren't. But you can cut one half of the nail at a time or work from one side to the other if you follow my other suggestion. Just soak your feet in warm water for twenty minutes before you try to cut the nails, and you'll find that they won't be nearly as brittle or hard."

"In a pan or something?"

"Or in the bathtub. This particular type of hot soak isn't trying to draw extra blood to the affected part like most of the others we've discussed (and have mentioned in this book), so it doesn't matter if your whole body is in the warm water."

Next time I saw Dorothy, her nails were trimmed back and much more comfortable.

"I did just as you told me," she said. "And I could cut them back all right. But the thick part still rubbed on my shoe a little, so I thought maybe I could file it down while it was soft. And that worked just fine. Maybe you can add that suggestion when you talk to other patients."

Or write for them, which is what I'm doing now.

THE GIST OF THIS CHAPTER

Probably the change most people fear most with the accumulation of the years is loss of memory. Yet many of the disturbing lapses and periods of confusion which plague people over sixty disappear when they simply drink plenty of noncaffeine-containing liquids. Other memory lapses stem from electrical seizure-type activity in the brain and yield readily to medicines such as Dilantin which do not dull your brain or change your functioning in any harmful way. Still others stem from partially plugged arteries leading to the brain, and yield to such simple remedies as aspirin and weight control, or in more serious cases to an operation which you can have with very little discomfort or disability.

Many of the problems of over-sixty stem from lack of hormones. Vaginitis, brittle bones, bowed back and undue wrinkling of the skin fall into this group. Although hormone creams available without a prescription can help these conditions, tablets usually prove cheaper and more convenient in the long run. You need to get a prescription for these from your doctor, partly because all hormones increase tumor risks slightly, but the over-all benefits outweigh this hazard whenever hormone lack is sufficiently severe to cause substantial complaints.

Sluggish circulation and unduly dry heated air cause most of the complaints which make winters tougher as the years go by. A snugly warm torso, plenty of liquids, activities in the outdoor air, and measures to humidify the indoors generally make cold weather much easier to bear. If you get cold hands or feet in spite of these measures, warm up with heat applied to the thighs or upper arms instead of directly to the affected part.

Digestive misery at night in the later years often comes from a hiatus hernia and yields to blocks under the head of the bed, weight reduction and occasionally antacids.

Thickened nails soften in warm water and can be cut off or filed with inexpensive equipment available in any drug store.

12

How to Control Skin Allergies, Rashes, and Infections

Skin trouble is an assault by four horsemen: itching, soreness, aggravation, and pain. Yet I have seen patients who endured this misery for years without even seeking relief. Such futile suffering! Most of these victims could cure themselves in their own homes with almost no expense, if they only knew what measures to take. The rest could almost always get at least temporary relief from home measures. Yet I have seen my good Minnesota patients itching and squirming without attempting to take these easy steps toward relief.

HOW TO FIGHT SKIN IRRITATIONS AND ALLERGIES

Chemical irritation causes many more visits to a skin specialist's office than any one skin disease. You can very frequently soothe those irritations right in your own home, with little or no expense. Furthermore, you can often discover what substances cause your trouble and eliminate them for permanent cure.

No matter what harsh chemical irritates your skin, you get the same complaints and changes, and need the same home remedies. Even if you mistake some other skin disease for skin sensitivity, properly chosen measures will usually prove highly effective, or at least harmless. Whenever you have skin irritation which is not so severe as to drive you to a doctor for powerful prescription aid, try these soothing remedies:

Weeping or blistered skin. Home remedies for blistered or weeping sores usually prove worthwhile unless pussy matter or thick, crumbling crusts point toward impetigo or similar infection. Wet applications rather than lotions or ointments are the safest home treatment for irritation-caused weeping, blisters, or cracks.

Soothing soaks. Two tablespoonfuls of Burow's solution to one pint of water at room temperature is the best remedy. Boric acid solution, one tablespoonful of powder to the pint, is second best for adults (but is not safe for children). A level teaspoonful of table salt to one pint of water or full strength cow's milk makes a satisfactory soak if you have nothing else on hand. If the dermatitis involves easily immersed parts such as hands, feet, or elbows, soak for 10 to 15 minutes at least four times daily. For other body parts, apply cloths wet with soothing solution for twenty minutes at least four times a day. With very severe rashes, you may want to use these measures still more frequently.

Skin-healing baths. Severe itching of widespread body parts calls for oatmeal baths. These usually give relief for eight hours or so, and speed healing of almost any type of dermatitis. Follow these directions:

> Boil two cups of slow-cooking oatmeal in two quarts of water for fifteen minutes. Fill your bathtub halfway with moderately warm water. Hold a piece of light cotton or fairly fine cheesecloth over the bathtub and pour the oatmeal into it. A light cotton sack or bag works very well. The cloth should strain the oatmeal out and allow the fluid to drain through into the tub. Gather the edges of the cloth and tie above the oatmeal with string. Now get into the tub. Use the oatmeal bag as a washcloth to pat the worst itching areas, and slosh it around in the bath water at intervals. Soak in the soothing solution for about 10 minutes.

Colloid baths. If your skin eruption seems likely to last more than a few days, you can get the benefit of oatmeal baths without the bother by using the purified oatmeal colloid, sold in your drugstore under the trade name "Aveeno." Use two cupfuls to a tub of water, and soak yourself for 20 minutes as often as your complaints require.

Soothing measures for red or raw skin eruptions. Skin irritations which are too mild to blister or crack usually yield to lotions or pastes. Most patchy, itching eruptions fall in this group.

Lotion. You can get zinc oxide lotion, which is very soothing for most skin lesions, without a prescription. Buy a small bottle of glycerin at the same time for use in removing cakes or crusts left by the lotion at the end of the day.

Pastes and ointments. If the irritated area is dry, scaly, or harsh-feeling, pastes and ointments work better than lotion. Lassar's paste requires no prescription, and is very soothing. Boric acid or zinc oxide ointments also help mildly irritated skin.

Cortisone creams. As this edition goes to press, the Food and Drug Administration has just released cortisone creams for nonprescription use. Cortisone has exactly the same action on your skin as the natural inflammation-fighting hormones made in your adrenal gland. It quickly became the most widely used and most effective prescription remedy for skin ailments after its introduction twenty years or so ago. What a blessing to have this potent preparation available as a home remedy today!

Although cortisone will also be sold in ointments and lotions, I recommend the cream because more of the active ingredient soaks into your skin where it can do some good. Cortisone is expensive, so it is important to get the most out of each dab. If you put a small amount on your skin and let it warm up to body temperature for a minute or so, it will spread several times as far. Only the portion of cream in actual contact with your skin does any good, so this approach helps cut costs without harming effectiveness.

Cortisone helps most skin irritations and allergies, and cuts down the misery from cold sores and virus infections. It does *not* help and may actually substantially *hurt* bacterial infections such as impetigo, infected scrapes and sores, boils, furuncles and pimples. Cortisone soaks into your system through the skin, and should not be used on large body areas. It impairs healing of cuts and burns, and should therefore never be used on any form of injury (including sunburn). If you use it properly, though, it will work wonders for localized irritations and allergic reactions. Two or three applications a day usually take out the itch immediately and heal the rash in a few days. Of course, you will have more trouble when you quit if your skin is still exposed to the original irritation or allergen, but you really don't need to suffer while you try to identify and eliminate the cause of your problem.

Home correctives for common skin sensitivities. You can usually cure skin irritation for good by using suitable substitutes for the substances that have been causing your trouble. The big trick is to identify the troublemakers. Keep track of when the rash flares and fades and watch what objects come in contact with the affected area. Then decide which might be offenders by keeping these points in mind:

1. Dermatitis usually flares within 24 hours of contact with the offending irritant. However, the abruptness of the flare does not mean that it occurs immediately after contact. One of my good farm women, for instance, developed a rash that itched and burned abruptly almost every evening after supper. When we finally discovered the source of her difficulty, it proved to be allergy to the chicken mash she spread by hand every morning, twelve to eighteen hours before the rash flared.

2. Dermatitis often develops suddenly from exposure to a substance that you have used previously without harmful effects. One of my patients had been in the baking trade for 24 years before he developed a rash, which we nevertheless proved was due to flour. A great many patients who learn the cause of their trouble only after several visits to a doctor say: ''Well, I

would have figured that out for myself, only I've used the same stuff for years without trouble.''

3. Dermatitis usually starts in the general vicinity of the spot touched by the offending substances, but there are several notable exceptions. The thick skin of the palm of the hand seldom becomes inflamed, so that inflammation of the back of the hand, wrist and lower arms often occurs from substances most of whose contact is with the palm. Fingernail polish frequently causes inflammation of the eyelids. Any dermatitis which becomes severe can spread far beyond the area of actual chemical irritation.

Let's see how these principles have helped several skin sufferers:

1. A housewife found that her blistered hands got worse every Friday. Since she cleaned house on Thursday, she soon traced her trouble to furniture polish.

2. A printer's face bumps got almost well by Monday morning, became troublesome again during the week. He ultimately found that he was sensitive to the brand of soap his boss provided.

3. A bank clerk whose hobby was photography came to work every Monday morning with red, raw hands until he learned that his skin reacted to one of the chemicals he used in his weekend darkroom work.

All of these victims cured themselves by applying the simple facts about skin sensitivity. Couldn't you do the same?

SPECIFIC SKIN IRRITATIONS

Some eruptions due to sensitive skin are so common that you can take a short cut to quick cure if you know about them. Here are specific directions for spotting and curing these common skin sensitivities:

Soap-burnt hands. Dry, rough, cracking skin on the hands usually comes from soap or detergents. More severe weeping, or blistering eruption of the backs or sides of the fingers and hands may also be due to soap. Ideal solution: avoid doing dishes, laundry, or floorscrubbing, at least until the rash is clear. Second best: wear lined rubber gloves or a pair of white cotton gloves with rubber gloves over them until your skin is clear. For continued protection, try a silicone protective lotion or cream such as Covicone, which you can get at any drugstore without a prescription. Apply three times a day for one week, twice a day for one week, and daily thereafter. Most patients find this almost as effective as rubber gloves and much less clumsy. For handwashing, super-bland detergents like pHisoderm work well. Nonperfumed bland soap like Ivory or Swan may prove safe after your hands have thoroughly healed.

Itching scalp. If itching scalp plagues you, or if you have a rash along the tops or backs of the ears and on your neck, shampoo chemicals may be at fault. One way to find out: clean your hair with the raw egg method for one month.

Egg shampoo. Beat two or three raw eggs, wet the hair with warm water, and rub in the beaten eggs thoroughly with the tips of your fingers. Rinse thoroughly with lukewarm water. Follow with a vinegar rinse, made from one teaspoonful of white vinegar in one quart of lukewarm water. Brush thoroughly while the hair is drying.

Saponified coconut oil. If you have only a normal degree of itching, you might want to try a special form of liquid soap as a shampoo. Saponified coconut oil, obtained from any pharmacy, is much gentler, more effective, and cheaper than most commercial shampoos. Many of my patients find it highly satisfactory for regular scalp cleansing.

Laundry detergent rash. Dry, red-pepper-granule dermatitis of the back and upper arms is often due to laundry detergent. The clothing clings in these areas. Perspiration provides a perfect bridge for chemicals to cross in reaching the skin. You can cure this condition quickly by washing clothes in bland soap powder such as Ivory Snow and rinsing them three times in soft water.

Cosmetic rash. When I ask a lady with a skin rash about cosmetics, she usually says: "But I don't use any." Most people take simple beauty aids such as lipstick, cleansing cream, toilet water and nail polish for granted. Yet these quite commonly cause skin trouble. Most women with blemishes or rash should eliminate all beauty aids, perfumed soaps and shampoos, nail polish and deodorants for a two week period. If the rash clears, they should resume beauty aids one at a time with a week or more lag between new agents until they find the offenders. Usually, different brands or specially compounded cosmetics will fill the beauty bill without causing further trouble.

Workman's eruption. Most people encounter harsh chemicals of some sort in the course of their work. Cutting oils, cement dust, harsh solvents, and cleaning agents are the commonest offenders on a mile-long list. If you have skin trouble which improves during vacations, your work is probably responsible. Under workmen's compensation laws, your employer usually has to pay for any care you need, so you might as well see a doctor. Moreover, you need the doctor's certificate that work caused your trouble before you can settle your claim.

Rash from medicines. Probably the most common form of sensitive-skin rash which you can control with home measures stems from your attempts to get and keep well. Every kind of medicine from aspirin tablets and vitamin capsules to skin lotions and ointments can sometimes cause skin rash. You can control or avoid this difficulty by following these rules:

1. Whenever you get a rash, eliminate all self-prescribed or nonessential medicines, including vitamin pills, laxatives, sleeping pills, and aspirin. If your doctor has prescribed medicines which you should continue because of some serious condition, call him up and ask him whether there is any chance that the medicine could be causing your rash.

2. If an abruptly appearing rash persists for more than two weeks or gets worse in spite of treatment, eliminate all ointments and applications (including any your doctor has prescribed). Use Burow's solution soaks or cloths, which are always safe, to keep your disorder under control. If medications have been prolonging or aggravating your condition, you should note an improvement in two days.

3. Treat skin ailments more gently the worse they seem to be. Use milder soaks instead of stronger ointments for persistent or highly troublesome skin ailments. Over-strong medicines drive more patients to skin specialists than any single disease. You can frequently keep yourself from requiring expensive specialized services for this reason. Here are two instructive examples:

H. G. developed an itchy, reddish blotch on the back of his left hand. His druggist suggested 5% ammoniated mercury ointment. After a week the rash seemed somewhat worse, so H. G. bought some stronger ointment—10% ammoniated mercury. Two weeks later, H. G. went to his doctor with blistering and redness extending almost up to his left elbow, and some rash of the back of the right hand. Key step to quick cure: omitting any further ammoniated mercury ointment.

M. T. had always used Whitfield's ointment for his athlete's foot, with excellent results. When he developed an unusually severe case with open cracks between his toes and burning blisters, he figured Whitfield's would do the trick. It burned like fire in the open cracks, but M. T. used it anyway. After ten days, his feet were so bad that he couldn't get to work any longer. On his wife's advice he switched to Burow's solution soaks. In two days, he was virtually well.

HOW TO CONTROL SKIN INFECTIONS WITH SIMPLE HOME CARE

You can control many small skin infections with simple home remedies and care. Ingrown hairs, boils, beginning infection beside the fingernail, mild festering, athlete's foot, and scabies frequently yield to proper home treatment. Here are several pointers for recognizing and dealing with these common problems:

Boils, ingrown hair, and infected sores. With a little help, your body can almost always fight off the germs that cause boils and minor skin infections. It does this by pouring germ-devouring white blood cells into the area. These white blood cells soon pile up in the form of pus and matter, which works to the skin surface. You can aid this natural method of body defense in several important ways:

1. Hot soaks or wet cloths. Heat helps to open up blood vessels in the infected area, lets more germ-devouring white blood cells get to the scene and makes infections come to a head much more quickly. If the sore is on a hand or foot where you can soak it, put the whole part down in water as hot as is completely comfortable (about 112 degrees, measured with a candy thermometer). Otherwise use a towel that's folded to six or eight thicknesses and dipped in hot water. Wring out the excess water and cover with a dry towel or piece of plastic. Switch to a freshly-dipped towel as often as necessary. Whether you soak or use cloths, continue the heat for 20 minutes at least four times a day.

2. How to open a pointed up sore. Pus or matter works its way toward the surface of your skin. It usually takes a day or two to stretch the skin and burst through. Once you can see yellow or white pus welling up in an infected sore, you can speed healing by opening it. The transparent skin at the point of a sore is dead tissue anyway, and ultimately will give way.

The best home method for opening a sore is with a flamed needle. First, clean the sore and the nearby skin with rubbing alcohol. Then pass the needle through a flame several times. Let the needle cool without touching anything. Hold the needle almost level with the skin. Push the tip along just under the point of the sore, but always within the transparent area. Lift up to break through the skin. Let the pus well up, perhaps pressing *very gently* on the area. Do not try to squeeze the pus out—more hot soaks will draw it out more safely and comfortably. Clean the surrounding skin again with alcohol. Put on a bandage. Use further hot soaks, right through the bandage.

3. Favor the infected part. You can help to heal an infection and limit its spread simply by resting the part. If you have any festering sore, every muscle you move in the vicinity milks some germs into the surrounding area. A big bandage that holds the part still and reminds you not to use it will speed your recovery a great deal. If bandaging isn't practical, favor the infected part as much as you can.

4. Germicidal cleansing. After each soak or at least four times a day, you should wipe off the whole area surrounding any infected sore with rubbing alcohol. At least once a day, you should definitely take a thorough shower with antiseptic-containing surgical soap such as Gamophene, obtainable at any drugstore without prescription. If the sore is located in your armpit or in another area where skin surfaces rub together, apply 5% ammoniated mercury ointment, which also requires no prescription, to the surrounding area twice a day. These precautions will help to keep the hordes of still-potent germs which stream out with the pus from infecting other nearby skin glands and perpetuating your problem. To cite a case:

"I've had so many boils in my armpits," Mrs. Lindell complained. "Eight or ten every year now, for the past twelve years."

Mrs. Lindell had tried countless kinds of medicine. She had given up deodorants and stopped shaving her armpits. Still she suffered misery from her boils. A program based on germicidal cleansing stopped all that. Mrs. Lindell washed her armpits thoroughly with surgical soap and wiped them with rubbing alcohol three times a day. Only one more boil appeared. While it was draining, she smeared 5 per cent ammoniated mercury ointment on all of the skin in the area to keep germs from getting into nearby glands. She washed her armpits with alcohol six times a day. From that time forth, she never had another boil.

Infection around a fingernail. Infections at the margin of the fingernails cause a great deal of pain. You can often stop such an infection for yourself without a doctor's help by prompt action.

Hot soaks. As soon as infection causes redness, throbbing pain, and slight swelling at the base or side of the nail, you should start using hot soaks. Soak the whole finger for twenty minutes at least four times a day in water which is as hot as you can stand without burning (112 degrees). This helps to draw the infection and get it ready to drain.

Drainage. You can often drain an infection around the fingernail before it starts to point up. Immediately after a hot soak, work the tip of a small scissors blade gently under the cuticle beside your infection. Gently lift the tip straight up to pull the cuticle away from the underlying nail. Work it in a little farther, and lift again. Repeat until matter wells up, or until further manipulation becomes painful. Do this every time you soak the finger for a day or so. If a drop or two of pus or matter does not drain out before two days have passed, best see a doctor.

Prevention. Housewives get eight times as many infections around the fingernails as office workers. The whole family's mouth germs wind up in the dishwater where they get a perfect whack at mother's fingers. This is one risk any woman can easily avoid. Just rinse your hands in a fresh stream of water for a few seconds after you dump the dishpan.

How to cure athlete's foot with home measures. You can usually control athlete's foot for yourself, without a doctor's aid. Itching, cracking, and peeling between the toes usually come from simple athlete's foot. Small blisters filled with cloudy fluid may spread to the base of the toes and the instep. Here's how to rid yourself of this disease:

Soaks. Heal open blisters or cracks with soaks before you use ointment on your athlete's foot. Potassium permanganate works well. It stains, so use an old basin or pot for soaking. Crush a five grain tablet thoroughly and dissolve it in one quart of water. Be sure the tablet is completely dissolved, because undissolved fragments will burn your skin. Soak your feet ten minutes every two hours. The soaks will turn your toenails brown, but this is a harmless color change. Permanganate tablets are very poisonous, so keep them in a safe place and flush leftover supplies down the toilet when you are well. Two to four days of soaking usually does the trick.

Ointments. If you have no open blisters or cracks, or if you have healed them with soaks, undecenylic acid ointment is your best bet. Apply it twice daily for at least one week after signs of athlete's foot have disappeared. In a few cases, undecenylic acid fails. Then you can use half strength Whitfield's ointment. Do not use full strength Whitfield's, which is too strong for many people's skin.

If ointments cause irritation, or if your condition fails to improve, see your doctor.

Sock sterilization. Athlete's foot germs can live for several months nestled in shoe leather or between the threads of your socks. By sterilizing your socks after each wearing and changing them every day, you can usually keep athlete's foot from coming back. The water you use in your own washing machine or in a self-help laundry is not hot enough to kill these germs. Either brief boiling or a trip to a commercial laundry (which uses water at 180 degrees) makes socks safe.

Measures to avoid reinfection. Once you know that you are susceptible to athlete's foot, you can save yourself a lot of misery by taking steps to avoid reinfection. Be sure that everyone in your household with even a trace of athlete's foot takes treatment at once. Take special precautions when you use a public shower or bath. Dry well between your toes: that prevents nine cases out of ten. If hazard is very high, as in the men's shower at work, use foot clogs and rub your feet with alcohol just before drying.

Psoriasis. The scaly, dry patches of psoriasis show up most frequently on the elbows, knees, and at the hairline. Fortunately, this unsightly state does not disfigure the face or cause unbearable itching and discomfort. Most victims have had trouble since their teens, and have asked doctors about the condition often enough to know exactly what is wrong with them and that no lasting cure is presently available. However, these simple home techniques usually give considerable improvement:

Ultraviolet ray. If your psoriasis tends to get better in the summertime, you will probably improve with ultraviolet ray baths. You will get the best results with an ultraviolet lamp which has a quartz tube rather than a glass one, since the most beneficial rays cannot pass through glass. A glass sunlight bulb is better than nothing, though. Several of my patients are in the habit of taking a sunbath while shaving and performing their morning toilet, which helps to make the treatments regular and still saves considerable time. If you go this route, be sure to keep the lamp and wires well away from both your body and the plumbing. Any electric appliance should be used with great care in the bathroom. During the summer, you can replace lamp treatments with natural sun baths.

Ultraviolet through tar ointment. One of the most effective measures for most psoriasis victims is the combination ointment-ultraviolet treatment. For this treatment, spread a thin coat of Taralba ointment over the scaly patches of psoriasis, then take a sunbath treatment right through the ointment. Either natural sunlight or ultraviolet light does well.

Ointment alone. A few psoriasis victims find that they get worse in the summertime or after sunbathing. These people should carefully protect themselves from sun, coating their psoriasis sores with a sunscreen lotion like Sundown when protection with clothing is not practical. An ordinary tar ointment helps most smoldering lesions. Very thick, heaped up plaques sometimes respond to a thorough mixture of three parts Taralba with one part Whitfield's ointment. Tegrin and Mazon ointments are good trade preparations.

Bland measures. When psoriasis shows signs of becoming rapidly worse, with new spots appearing, old spots spreading, or considerable itching and discomfort, you should usually omit any tar, or ultraviolet treatment. At this stage, zinc oxide ointment and soothing oatmeal baths often help. Your doctor's advice will prove worthwhile, too.

The itch. Diseases sometimes undergo an abrupt change, sometimes for no apparent reason. That's what happened to the "seven year itch," and it happened very abruptly soon after the last edition of this book came out. The former editions talked about lines of tiny blisters, especially on the finger webs as characteristic of this disease. But if you get the itch today—which you well might because there's been a worldwide epidemic in the past few years—it won't look anything like the "old fashioned" type. The most likely part of your body to be involved today is the genital area, with the buttocks, armpits, abdomen and chest next likely in that order. You may still find a trail of tiny blisters at the onset of any one episode, but you'll have to be quick—the modern form gets to the crusted sore stage in a matter of an hour or two, and tends to have much more widespread redness and puffiness to obscure the picture. In fact, this new form of the disease often baffles even a trained physician. There's only one reasonably reliable tip-off: if your trouble is "the itch," other members of the family almost always come down with it within ten days or so. No matter what the itching areas look like, if the whole household has them the odds strongly favor scabies as the source.

If family involvement and the appearance or distribution of the itching suggest scabies, start your treatment with a prolonged hot bath and thorough soap-and-washcloth scrubbing. Follow immediately with a chin-to-toe application of 25 per cent benzyl benzoate emulsion or benzyl benzoate-DDT lotion, either obtainable at any drugstore. You'll usually need some help to be sure your whole back and other areas are covered. Repeat the application again the next morning *but not on any later occasion* (extra repetitions often cause skin irritation and dermatitis). To avoid reinfection, check all other members of the family, and treat anyone with suspicious scratch marks or lesions simultaneously. Change to clean, hot-water laundered underwear and clothing, and either hot-water launder, dry clean or iron (ironing kills the mites, too) all clothes and bedclothes.

If itching continues after this treatment, it is usually due to skin irritation from the medicines and mildly infected scratch marks rather than from continued scabies. Starch or oatmeal baths (see above) generally give quick relief.

As an alternative program, slightly more expensive but much easier and less irritating to the skin, try Kwell cream or lotion. Bathe and dry thoroughly, then apply Kwell to all affected areas and do not wash off for 24 hours. One application usually does the trick.

Head lice, body lice, crab lice, and bedbugs. Many years ago, my father (who was an eminent skin specialist) examined an obviously wealthy, superbly groomed woman who complained of an itching scalp. He could find nothing wrong, so he advised her to come back in a week without washing her hair. The cause of her misery literally galloped into view, and he exclaimed:

"Madam, you are lousy!"

Ignoring her stunned expression, he instructed that everyone in the household be treated at once, all the bedclothing boiled or ironed and so forth.

"But you don't understand," the patient said. "I have the most crucial house guests—how can I ever tell the central committee of the D.A.R. that they may all have head lice?"

I don't know whether anything helped this poor woman bear up under her social anguish, but it might give her some comfort to know that her story has relieved a great many people from any feeling of shame at encountering lice. It happens in the best of families, no matter how clean and careful you might be.

For either head lice or crab lice (found in pubic hair and armpits) Kwell shampoo is a definitely superior treatment. It kills both the lice and their nits (eggs which adhere to the hair). One thorough application usually suffices. DDT powder or lotion also kills the lice, but to avoid recurrence you usually have to trim the hair quite short and comb it very carefully with a fine-toothed metal comb to remove all nits. For body lice or "cooties" Kwell cream or lotion works very well. If you don't actually see the lice but get insect bites on exposed body areas, check carefully for bedbugs. Caladryl or other soothing treatment suffices for the bites, but you may need anything from DDT to a professional exterminator to rid yourself of the problem.

LEISURE TIME SKIN ASSAULTS

From the hordes of pallid Easterners who stream into Minnesota's wide open spaces every year, it seems safe to assume that almost everyone is spending more time outdoors these days. At times, traffic to the far wilderness is almost bumper to bumper around the Fourth of July. Along with the extra fun, more outdoor life brings miseries like insect bites, poison ivy rash and sunburn. Believe me, the Land of Lakes has given home remedies for these ailments a thorough trial!

Bee sting. If you get hives or severe general reaction to bee sting, you should check with your doctor for special medicine you can carry around with you. Such allergic reactions to bee sting sometimes become more and more severe until they become really serious or even fatal. Ordinary bee sting, which causes pain and swelling only in the vicinity of the sting itself, responds well to home measures.

Knifetip scraping. Most people make the mistake of trying to grasp the stinger with their fingers or with tweezers when they suffer a bee sting. In the process, they squeeze on the poison sac at the outer end of the stinger and make their ultimate reaction much worse. You should remove the stinger by gentle scraping with the tip of a sharp knife.

Ammonia solution. Ammonia helps to neutralize the formic acid which makes bee stings and ant bites painful. Mix two teaspoonfuls of household ammonia with one glass of water and use as a soak or compress immediately, before the sting opening has a chance to seal. Wasp and yellowjacket stings also respond to ammonia.

Nerve numbing agents. Ointments and lotions which make the pain nerves in the area insensitive definitely lessen the discomfort you suffer from a bee sting. Surfacaine cream numbs surface nerves safely. The same pain-relieving ingredient is combined with a preparation which fights later swelling in the very useful Surfadil lotion. Your druggist sells both preparations without requiring a prescription.

Mosquito and other insect bites. Itching insect bites respond best to soothing and antihistamine-containing lotions. Caladryl lotion works fairly well. Surfadil is very effective, too. If you do not have these on hand, a paste of bicarbonate of soda and water sometimes gives some comfort.

Poison ivy. The first time you get poison ivy, the rash usually develops up to 10 days or so after your exposure. Later attacks come on within a few hours. Ivy rash often spreads beyond the area of actual contact, but this spread results from the skin's sympathetic response to distant irritation instead of from contact with the blister fluid as many people think. You can break ivy blisters safely without spreading the irritation.

Unroofing blisters. You can usually make ivy dry up more quickly by taking the tops off of the blisters. Wipe the area with rubbing alcohol or clean it thoroughly beforehand. Use a flamed needle to open small blisters. Scissors and tweezers work best for taking the roofs off large fluid-filled pockets.

Soothing compresses. Mix two tablespoonfuls of Burow's solution, which you can get at any drug store without a prescription, with one glassful of lukewarm water. Wet cloths with this solution and apply to the itching areas. Cover with a layer of plastic sheeting or with a plastic refrigerator bag and leave in place for 30 to 45 minutes. Repeat four times daily.

Lotions. For milder forms of poison ivy or for healing cases, zinc oxide lotion is very soothing. For even faster results when the area involved is small, cortisone cream (see p. 158) usually dries up ivy in two to three days.

Sunburn. If you get a small patch of sunburn where your arm has hung out of the car window or where shirtsleeves have been shorter than the ones you were accustomed to, Surfacaine cream will give you a lot of relief. For any substantial body area, however, Surfacaine cannot be used. These measures deserve a try:

Double strength Burow's. Two-thirds cupful of Burow's solution with enough water to make one pint is good for sunburn. If a wide area is involved, you may want to use tablets or powders to mix a larger quantity. Ask your druggist for directions. However you prepare the solution, wet several light towels, handkerchiefs, or strips of sheeting with it and apply to the burned area. In severe burns, you will probably want to use such applications for one hour out of each two, while milder burns may respond to 20 minute applications two or three times a day.

Calamine lotion. When you cannot use wet applications or for milder sunburn, try calamine lotion. However, be sure that you get plain rather than phenolated lotion, and buy a small bottle of glycerin to remove lotion crusts.

Ice for Sunburn. If you can freeze a sunburnt area just as the skin reaction is occurring, you can often cut down the damage quite substantially. The most dramatic demonstration of this I've seen occurred in my own family, where one of the youngsters was becalmed on a sunbathed lake at the very start of the season and reached shore just as her skin was starting to get red. We were camped far from any source of extra ice but used what we had on one side of her back. The other side blistered and became very sore, but the treated side hardly even got red. The technique is given in detail under "the instant freeze for burns" in the next chapter.

BLACKHEAD AND PIMPLE PROBLEMS

Don't treat all "zits" as acne. Raised reddish spots on the face and shoulders often come from dermatitis (see above), especially if the spots come up very quickly, are itchy instead of tender, and feel fairly pliable and soft. Dermatitis clears without being picked or squeezed and does not leave pits or scars. Mild acne may not drain or scar, but at least some of the pimples usually come to a head.

The outer layers of skin are made up of dead cell shells. Minor chemical changes, resulting at least partly from diet, can let those shells heap up around the openings of your skin's oil glands. This plugs the oil glands and causes blackheads, pimples or skin cysts. You can attack this chain of events at several points.

Diet. Whether or not you "are what you eat," your food choices have a lot to do with skin texture. Nuts and nut products, including peanut butter, and carbonated beverages seem to be the biggest factors in producing pimples. Although some recent studies seem to disagree, most of my patients also do better without chocolate and fried or fatty foods (including potato chips, french fries and fried-center hamburgers).

Vitamin A. Large quantities of Vitamin A help to condition your skin cells. The change increases oil gland openings and makes blackheads or pimples much less likely to appear. Use 50,000 unit tablets three times a day. Effects may be rather gradual, so it takes about a six-week trial to tell whether you are getting any help. There have been some reports that very prolonged (many years) use of this Vitamin can produce kidney stones, so check with your doctor before extending your treatment time beyond one year.

Skin-thinning soaps. Especially for acne on the shoulders and back, Lava soap or Mechanic's grit soap often works wonders. Rub the cake directly on the areas usually affected to thin the skin slightly and open up oil pores. Once a pimple has started this treatment does no good. Don't rub on the tender, raised pimples. Several showers a week with firm friction on the nontender affected areas will usually keep shoulders and back pimples under fairly good control.

Drying lotions. If you can shrink your skin slightly with a drying lotion, the pores and oil gland openings gape open. This prevents pimples and blackheads from getting a start. White lotion U.S.P. is the standard preparation, which any druggist can supply. Acnomel and several other trade preparations combine drying lotions with pimple-covering pigment.

Perhaps because of the cover-up feature, most people do not use these lotions correctly. The idea is to open up skin glands and keep pimples or blackheads from forming in the first place, not to treat already-formed pimples. You should therefore apply the lotion to the entire affected area (usually the face and base of the neck) rather than to the pimples and blackheads themselves. Wash the area thoroughly at bedtime, apply the lotion and leave it in place until morning, when you can wash it off again.

Blackhead squeezing. Get a blackhead squeezer for about 25 cents at the nearest drugstore. This has small, spoon-shaped portions at each end with a smooth-rimmed hole in the center. Wipe off the area with rubbing alcohol and allow to dry. Place either the larger or the smaller hole (whichever matches the size of the blackhead best) directly over the blackhead. Press the squeezer straight into the skin, without allowing it to slide or skid along the skin at all. The contents of the blackhead should pop through the hole like a little white worm before the pressure reaches an uncomfortable level.

If a blackhead will not pop with the amount of pressure you can readily tolerate, you can soften its top with warm, wet cloths for ten minutes. Hot towels or "facial saunas" increase oil gland activity and make the underlying condition worse, though, so you should use them only when other methods fail.

Pimple picking. As long as a pimple is hard, you should never squeeze or pick it. The worst acne pustules and pitted scars result from squeezing a pimple before the skin covering has thinned out, so that the pus has no way to burst but inward. Most pimples will point up in a whitehead, with a thinned-out bit of transparent skin confining the drop of pus underneath.

Some remain red in the center but become very soft and loose at the drainable spot. Until one or the other of these changes occurs, you should not pick or pinch at a pimple.

To open a pointed-up pimple, first pass the point of a needle through the flame of a match two or three times. Put the needle on the edge of your kitchen counter with the point hanging untouched in open air. Wipe off the pimple with rubbing alcohol. Hold the needle parallel with the skin and insert its point from the edge of the whitehead or central softness toward its center. Pull straight up away from the skin, breaking through a few skin cells. Press gently with a blackhead squeezer to see whether pus will break through, and if not pick slightly deeper. If you cause either oozing or flow of blood, stop and make gentle pressure through a cotton ball or gauze pad until the bleeding stops (usually three to four minutes without peeking). Do not squeeze pus through a bleeding surface—open blood vessels give the germs in pus a ready passage into your system, sometimes causing infection to spread.

Antibiotics and other prescription care. Very deep or painful pustules sometimes call for antibiotics. X-ray treatment or surface freezing may cause great improvement. Board-like or pitted skin can sometimes be thinned by surgical sandpapering. These measures are expensive and long drawn out, but they may be much better than the psychologic and social effects of permanently scarred and disfigured skin. Your family doctor should be able to give you some help with severe pimples, or to help you to locate a specialist who can give greater aid.

IMPETIGO, INFECTED SCRAPES AND OTHER SURFACE INFECTIONS

Since the last edition of this book came out, the F.D.A. has released Bacitracin Ointment for nonprescription use. With this very effective string in your home treatment bow, you can sometimes now safely try to cure yourself before seeing a doctor with these ailments.

Impetigo starts with an irregularly shaped blister filled with cloudy fluid. Since it itches intensely, you may scratch the top off the blister before you recognize what is going on. Thus the lesion may look like a crusted sore instead of a blister when you first look at it. The crust usually seems thick and crumbly rather than hard and adherent like an ordinary scab.

If you have any youngsters below the age of three in the household, impetigo deserves prompt prescription care. The disease spreads readily in the household, and can become very serious or even fatal in the very young. Adults and older children can try home care if there is no danger of spread to infants.

With impetigo or any other surface infection (other than herpes, as described above), try Bacitracin Ointment four times a day. Take a shower every day to remove germs from still-unaffected areas of the skin. Boil or send to a commercial laundry (where the water is generally hotter than at home or in a laundromat) all underclothing and bedclothing. Since spread from person to person generally occurs by way of the hands, frequent handwashing and perhaps an after-washing rinse with rubbing alcohol is worthwhile.

Perhaps I am prejudiced in favor of Bacitracin Ointment, since my father did some of the original research which produced it. In my experience, though, it has proved very effective and free of side effects.

13

Updated Home Care for
Everyday Injuries

Here in Minnesota it's always open season for injuries. Skiing sprains, fishermen's falls, campers' ax cuts, and hunters' wounds keep the bandage business brisk. Home accidents which you might expect in any of the 50 states keep Minnesotans hopping, too. Bruises, strains and sprains, scrapes, cuts, and burns add up to a considerable burden of misery which well-chosen home measures can greatly relieve. Even the smallest scratch involves some risk of infection, too: home measures often ward off serious trouble by keeping wounds clean.

HOME REMEDIES FOR BRUISES, STRAINS, AND SPRAINS

You can keep down swelling, disability, and pain in bruises, strains, and sprains by taking proper home measures immediately after you get hurt. You can speed your recovery from such injuries with proper care. You need no special equipment or expensive materials to accomplish these ends: you probably have everything you need in your house right now.

How to make sure that you don't have a fracture. Suppose that you fall or bump yourself or twist your ankle. Before you decide upon home measures, you want to be sure that you have no broken bones. Here are the usual rules of thumb:

1. Even slight tenderness over the small bones of the fingers, hands, wrist, toes, foot, ankle, and nose may mean fracture.

2. Even slight tenderness over a bone that has been wrenched instead of struck may mean fracture. Bony tenderness in a twisted ankle or wrist has to come from pulled ligaments or from wrenched-loose bone. Only X-rays can reliably distinguish.

3. Changes in body contour other than simple swelling at the site of injury almost always mean fracture. Compare the injured extremity with its

mate, especially with regard to bony knobs or prominences. Any difference between the two sides calls for a doctor's evaluation.

4. If jolting or compression conveyed along the shaft of the injured bone causes pain, fracture is almost always present. When you press straight back on your breastbone, for instance, rib fractures at the side of your chest usually hurt. Thumping on the bottom of the heel usually causes pain in any fracture from above the ankle to the hip. Thumping on the elbow or outstretched fist in such a way as to send a jolt straight up along the arm bones has similar effect. Naturally, you should use this maneuver only as a final check if no other evidence points strongly toward fracture.

5. Any pain in the middle of your back after a fall deserves a phone call to your doctor *before you attempt to get up.*

Two further cautions: Don't regard ability to move a part or put your weight on it as proof that the bones are intact. And don't assume that the part that hurts the worst is the one most seriously injured. If you have a serious fall or accident, run your hands over each extremity and each rib, check for tenderness in your abdomen and neck, and test for painless motion in each part of your spine before you try to get up.

How to hold down damage from a bruise, strain, or sprain. For the first 24 hours or more, the key remedies for any bruising or wrenching injury are cold applications, snug elastic bandages, gravity-aided blood drainage, and rest. Your aim at this stage is to prevent the leakage of fluid or blood from damaged blood vessels in the bruised or torn body parts. Cold shrinks those blood vessels, elastic bandages and gravity-aided blood drainage cut leakage from them, and rest lets them seal off leaks thoroughly and quickly. Here are specific techniques for applying these basic remedies:

Ice application. With ordinary bumps and bruises, you should apply ice immediately. Wrap an ice cube or a handful of crushed ice in a towel or washcloth and moisten the cloth with cold water. Apply directly to the injured area for ten to fifteen minutes. Do not put ice into direct contact with your skin, since it will sometimes cause a frost burn.

Ice bags. For sprained or strained ankles, large bruises, and other injuries to areas as large as the palm of your hand, you will probably find a padded ice bag the most convenient way to apply cold. An inexpensive plastic refrigerator bag works very well. Fill it about half way with crushed ice, add two or three tablespoonfuls of cold water, double or twist the open end and seal with a rubber band, and wrap the whole arrangement with a moist towel. Apply directly to the injured area for 10 to 15 minutes.

Cold cloths or soaks. If the injured area is larger than the palm of your hand or if you have no ice available, you may want to use cold cloths or soaks. Water fresh from the tap should be cold enough, even in areas where the pipes aren't as deeply buried as ours in the North Country. Soak the entire injured part for twenty to thirty minutes, adding fresh cold water or ice occasionally to keep the water cold. If you want to use cold cloths, fold a towel over until it is six or eight layers thick, dip it in cold water, wring it partially dry and apply to the injured part. Change as often as necessary to keep it cold. Continue for half an hour.

Elastic bandages. You can often keep down swelling in an injured extremity by putting on an elastic bandage. The rubber-containing brands work best. Wind the bandage in a spiral with about half its width overlapping on each turn. It should be snug, not too tight: if you apply it stretched about half as far as possible, you will find it just snug enough. When you have finished with your elastic bandage, wash it in lukewarm water with mild soap and dry it by draping it in loops along a line, so that the whole weight of the bandage does not stretch one end of it out of shape.

Gravity-aided blood drainage. If blood goes definitely downhill in the veins which lead from an injured area to the heart, injured vessels have less pressure and congestion in them. This reduces seepage of fluid and blood.

You can provide this kind of gravity-aided drainage in several ways. With bruises, strains and sprains of the hand or wrist, a properly adjusted sling will hold your hand at shoulder height in the daytime. When you lie down, let your hand rest on your chest and adjust a couple of pillows under your elbow and upper arm. You can improve drainage from a hurt foot or ankle by placing two pillows under the lower leg. Keep the lower leg level with the floor, since tight leaders in the back of the knee block circulation slightly if the leg is propped up straight.

Rest. Almost every athlete I know thinks that he can cut down trouble from a bruise or sprain if he works the injured part right away. Unfortunately, just the opposite is true: exercise makes any bruising or rending injury worse until swelling has reached its peak and started to subside, which usually takes about 24 hours. You can use splinting or adhesive strapping according to the techniques described in the next section as soon as you can get the necessary equipment together. Meanwhile, don't use the affected part any more than you can help.

How to speed recovery from a bruise, strain, or sprain. After swelling has reached its peak and started to subside, you need home remedies to help speed your body's processes of repair. You want to draw more circulating blood to the area, break up congestion and hold torn tissues steady in their proper places while they mend. Here are several effective techniques:

Heat. After swelling reaches its peak, which usually takes about 24 hours, heat helps more than cold. At this stage, you want to open up nearby blood vessels so that they can carry away the fluid and blood which leaked from the injured (but now sealed) vessels. Hot soaks or hot wet towels for 30 minutes three or four times a day benefit any bruise, strain, or sprain. As you add hot water or re-dip your towels, always check the temperature with your uninjured hand; otherwise, the treated part may become sufficiently accustomed to heat to let you burn yourself. A good many of our Minnesota housewives can be even more precise: after years of seeing how ladies with candy thermometers win more prizes at the state and county fairs, they've stormed the hardware stores for such equipment. Comes time for hot applications and they can keep the water at exactly 112 degrees, which is perfect!

Massage. One thing you have to give our farm families: each member will do almost anything for the others. Whenever anybody gets a bruise, strain, or sprain, they'll all pitch in to help heal it up faster. Massage definitely improves circulation and speeds healing with all these problems. Here's the exact technique for bruises or strains of the leg:

> Lie down with the injured part bared and arranged comfortably on two or more pillows. Have your helper powder the leg thoroughly from ankle to thigh with talc or bath powder. He should rub gently with the palm of the hand and with limp fingers, starting from midcalf level and stroking up toward the hip. Strokes should be gentle, rhythmic, and all in the same direction. Your helper should gradually increase the pressure applied at the center of each stroke, but should begin and end each stroke gently and smoothly throughout the treatment. Your helper can make his stroke as if your leg were a piece of clay he is shaping into a gracefully tapered vase. Massage should move closer and closer to the swollen, tender area, but should never quite reach it: your object is to improve circulation in the part, not to rub or work the injured area. Twenty minutes of stroking once a day usually speeds healing quite substantially.

Similar massage works well for injuries of the arm.

Strapping. You can brace most strained or sprained joints very effectively with adhesive strapping. If you have to put tape on a very hairy part, dry-shave the area first with a safety razor and a new blade. You will usually find that tape goes on best if you cut an approximate length and apply the middle first, allowing both ends to seek the exact sites at which they lie down most smoothly. Tape should always be laid on instead of put on under tension. If you want to pull a part in a given direction with tape, turn it that way and apply the tape without further pull. If tape tends to irritate your skin somewhat, apply a coat of tincture of benzoin and let it dry before putting on the adhesive. You can always make narrower strips from whatever width tape you have on hand by cutting a length, nicking the end, and tearing lengthwise. Here are the exact techniques you should use to strap each of the most common strains and sprains:

Stubbed small toe. All the toes except the big toe work together as a unit when you walk. If one of them gets hurt, you can make it much more comfortable by strapping the four smaller toes together. Cut four foot-long strips of half-inch adhesive tape. With the toes relaxed and in their natural position, slip the center of one strip between the big toe and its neighbor, with its sticky side toward the smaller toes, as close to the base of the toe as possible. Lay the upper end of the tape across the top of the toes, and smooth its loose end down along the side of your little toe and the sole of your foot. Lay the bottom end of the tape along the bottom of the toes so that it crosses the upper strip on the outer side of the little toe and ends on the top of your foot. Slip another strip of tape between the big toe and its neighbor. Overlap about half its width and run it parallel to the first strip. Continue in this fashion until all four strips have been applied. The last two or three strips will tend to cross at the ends of the toes instead of at the outer side of the foot, but this will remain comfortable so long as the tape is laid on instead of pulled tight.

Sprained big toe. You can strap your big toe all by itself. Cut three strips of half-inch tape each eight inches long. With the toe straight and relaxed, stick the middle of one strip fairly low down on the end of the toe. Direct the ends so that they will cross above the far toe joint and run up along the top of the foot. Apply the other strips back along the toe overlapping half their width, then gently lay two or three circular turns of tape around the toe itself.

Arch strain. Pain on the outer side of the foot after a wrenching injury usually comes from an arch strain. You can speed healing by taking the stretch off the injured ligaments and bracing them. One-inch adhesive works best. Cut three strips of tape about one foot long. Turn the foot and heel inward. Apply the middle of one adhesive strip diagonally across the outer side of the heel and bring the ends around so that one crosses the inner side of the foot just below the ankle bone and the other comes up over the arch. Apply the other two strips similarly, overlapping about half their width. Now cut three slightly longer strips of tape. Turn the front part of the foot outward as far as it will go. Apply the center of one adhesive strip to the sole of the foot just behind the base of your toes. Lead both ends up across the top of the foot and back around the arch. Apply the other two strips approximately parallel, overlapping about half their width at the start. Now apply circular strips of tape over the rest of the arch to make the whole dressing into a smooth, foot-covering sheet.

Strained or sprained ankle. So long as the most tender spot in a turned ankle is *below* instead of *at* the tip of the ankle bone, you probably have a sprain or strain instead of a fracture. Use three strips of one inch adhesive tape each about thirty inches long and a three inch elastic bandage for a satisfactory home dressing. Turn the foot sharply outward on the ankle. Apply the middle of one strip of tape across the bottom of the heel so that the ends lead up both sides of the ankle. If the shape of your leg does not permit a symmetrical, stirrup-like strapping, be sure that the end going up the outer side of your leg goes straight up, even if the other end tends to wind toward the front of the leg or around the foot. Apply the other two strips of tape more or less parallel and overlapping at the heel, and let their ends seek positions in which the tape lies down smoothly. Wrap the elastic bandage on top of the tape, starting with an anchor turn around the ankle, then taking alternate turns around the ankle and the arch, and then spiraling up the leg.

Strained or sprained thumb. When an accident bends your thumb back, the joint at its base usually gives. Hold this joint straight while you strap it. First put two strips of half inch tape lengthwise along the top of the thumb from tip to wrist. Cut five strips of half inch tape about one foot long. Place the middle of one strip across the palmar portion of the tip of the thumb. Direct the ends so that they will spiral up the thumb onto the back and the heel of the hand. Place further parallel strips overlapping up the thumb until the entire thumb is covered and the fan of tape from its base spreads to about half of the wrist. Two or three circular turns of adhesive around the wrist help to anchor the tape ends so that they will not curl up and come loose.

Strained or sprained finger. You can strap a mildly sprained finger with adhesive with the method just described by spiraling up from the tip and fanning out along the back of the hand. One or two strips of tape around the hand at the base of the fingers will anchor the tape ends.

Baseball fingers. For severely sprained fingers or fingers injured by a blow into the fingertip, the hairpin splint makes a very effective and comfortable dressing. You need a little flexible collodion (which you can buy without a prescription), some gauze roller bandage (preferably one inch wide), and one or two old fashioned U-shaped hairpins. Wind two layers of bandage on the finger as smoothly as possible. With a small pledget of cotton or an applicator stick, wet the bandage with collodion and allow to dry for two or three minutes. Shape the hairpin to the upper surface of the finger and hold it in place with two more layers of gauze. Moisten with collodion again. If you are planning to work with the injured hand, shape another hairpin to the front of the finger. Apply two more layers of gauze and wet with collodion. Apply more gauze and collodion until you have built a sturdy dressing, allowing each layer to dry thoroughly before applying the next. If you have trouble with the gauze coming loose, wind it diagonally in such a way that both ends are up on the palm of the hand where you can hold them until the collodion sets, then trim them off.

Strained or sprained wrist. You can strap a sprained wrist fairly effectively with the hand in the tipped-up position. First apply a strip of two inch adhesive along the top of the tipped-up wrist from the knuckles to the middle of the forearm. Cut three strips of one inch adhesive about two feet long. Apply the middle of one strip across the palm of the hand at the base of the fingers. Direct the ends so that they cross at the middle of the back of your hand and again in front of the wrist. Apply further strips with considerable overlap on the palm of the hand, but direct the ends to make the overlap decrease somewhat along the course of the tape. A two-inch elastic bandage gives an ideal finish to the dressing. Wind it around the wrist first, wind two or three turns alternately around the wrist and the hand, then spiral up the forearm. If an elastic bandage is not available, finish the dressing with two or three circular turns of tape around the midforearm.

Persistent discomfort in sprains or strains. An injured ligament should heal in ten to fourteen days. If discomfort continues after this time, strapping seldom does any good. At this point, you should switch to contrast baths. Bathe the whole part, not just the sore place. Soak the affected part in warm water (105°F.) for four minutes, in cold water (50°F.) for one minute, then back into the warm. Continue alternating, four minutes warm and one minute cold, for about 30 minutes. Always begin and end with warm.

Massage, as described above, is especially effective if performed immediately after a contrast bath.

Blown-up knee or elbow bursa. After unaccustomed activity or injury, you might abruptly develop a painful swelling at the front of your knee or above the point of your elbow. This generally comes from bleeding into a bursa, which is a smooth-walled collapsed sack (like an empty balloon with a few drops of oil in it). Bursas normally occur at friction points between muscle and tendon layers and act as bearings when adjacent structures rub against one another. If injury or strain breaks a tiny blood vessel inside a bursa, there is no pressure to help stop the bleeding until the entire bursa has filled. By that time, enough blood is in the space to keep the area sore for two or three weeks. If pain and swelling have reached a substantial level before you can start home treatment, you will be better off going to a doctor. He can draw out the blood with a needle and syringe and inject cortisone to keep down irritation. But if you start right away, home measures often do the trick.

Household treatment for this condition is just like that described for bruises. If you can chill the part right away, before much bleeding has occurred, you may stop hemorrhage immediately. A firm pressure dressing also helps, with a three-inch elastic bandage for the elbow or a four-inch one for the knee. Apply this in figure-eight style, with one loop above the joint and one below (crossing in the fold, not over the swollen bursa). By working up and down, you can cover the affected area with a firm, well-anchored bandage which will not separate at the crucial area when the extremity is bent, as a spiral bandage does.

Best continue cold applications two or three times a day and pressure bandages between for three days or so. Lukewarm soaks can be substituted for the cold applications thereafter, to speed absorption of the blood and aid healing.

Other bruising or wrenching injuries. Special home measures are very helpful for smashed fingers or toes, sprained knees, and sprained backs. Here's what to do about these common problems.

Mashed fingers or toes. A mashed finger or toe often shows a blue-black puddle of blood underneath the nail. This form of bruising causes severe discomfort because the accumulated blood presses on highly sensitive nerve endings. It also leads to loss of the nail unless the pressure is promptly relieved. First step is thorough cleanliness: wash your hands well and wipe off the affected finger with rubbing alcohol so that you will not get germs into the space underneath the nail while draining the blood out. Then follow one of these three methods:

Hot paper clip drainage. Unwind the first two turns of a metal paper clip and heat the free end to white heat with a cigarette lighter, gas flame or candle. Steady the injured finger against the tabletop and touch the hot paper clip end to the center of the blue-black area. If the blackish blood does not drain out, reheat the metal and apply it again until you burn a hole all the way through the nail (about 1/16 of an inch).

Knifetip drilling. Clean a sharp, pointed penknife blade and the injured finger thoroughly with rubbing alcohol. Steady the injured finger against a tabletop, and press the point of the knife gently into the center of the blue-black area. Twist the knifeblade clockwise and counterclockwise for ninety degrees or more, gradually increasing pressure. When you have drilled through the nail, blackish blood will ooze out of the first needlepoint-sized hole. Wipe away the blood with a freshly ironed handkerchief or sterile pad, and pick away at the margins of the hole with the knife point until it is as large as the eye in a small needle.

Nail margin peeling. A badly mashed finger may reaccumulate blood after the hole you burn or drill has sealed off. If so, the blood often works its way to the edge of the nail. Whenever there is a blue-black margin of skin at the edge of the nail, you will find that the easiest and most comfortable way to drain the puddled blood away is by peeling the discolored skin away from the nail edge with a blunt nail file. If the blood does not drain out during the peeling process, you will find that the skin layer inside the blue-black margin is dead like the top of a blister, and can be pierced and torn back with a flamed needle.

After-care. As long as blood seeps from a hole in or around the nail, keep a clean, dry bandage in place. If the nail begins to separate, trim the loose margins short with clippers so that they will not catch and tear the rest of the nail loose. As the new nail grows in, it will push the old one loose without pain or danger.

Sprained knees. As long as a sprained knee is sore and swollen, your best bet is to use cold compresses, hot towels, rest, and elastic bandaging. Cold helps most during the first 24 hours, as often as you can get around to it (but not more than one hour out of every two). Hot wet towels thereafter for half an hour three or four times a day often help. A severely sprained knee should keep you off your foot for several days either on crutches or strictly at home with only such walking as is necessary for self-care. A three- or four-inch elastic bandage helps a lot. Wrap the knee partially bent. Anchor the bandage with one or two turns below the knee, then run diagonally up the back of the knee, around the thigh and diagonally down the back of the knee. Use this above-and-below winding as you overlap each turn perhaps half the bandage width until the joint is firmly braced.

Healing sprains and trick knees. If your knees sometimes lock or give way, torn ligaments or cartilages are usually at fault. Even mild sprains leave ligaments weak and relaxed. In either case, you need to build knee-bracing muscle strength. Certain of your thigh muscles bridge the knee with what can become a sturdy, bracing girdle of muscle fibers. You can keep your knee completely stable even if one of its ligaments is completely torn away, by building tone in these muscles. Do this exercise three times a day for three weeks, and once daily thereafter:

> Sit in a straight chair with your leg stretched out straight in front of you. Set the muscles at the front of your thigh hard, pulling the kneecap up toward your hip, for five seconds. Keeping the muscle firm, slowly raise your heel about four inches off the floor. Hold the leg in this position for about five seconds. Let the heel down slowly, keeping the thigh muscles set. Relax the thigh muscle after another five seconds. After a five second rest, repeat. Continue for five to ten contractions.

How to cure back sprains and strains. Better than nine out of ten patients with low back strain severe enough to drive them to hospital care got complete relief with a program of rest, exercise, and postural training which you can closely mimic in your own home. Here are the five steps which many of my patients have used to move from back misery to permanent relief.

1. Rest in the jackknife position. Buy a piece of one inch plywood to fit between your coil or box springs and your mattress. If you have an innerspring mattress, place the plywood on top of it and obtain a cotton mattress to place on that. Saw across the plywood (or ask the lumberyard man to do so) about 30 inches from the top, and install hinges. Run one thickness of masking tape or cloth tape around the edges to avoid splinters in your fingers while making the bed. Raise the head end of the board to a 45-degree angle and prop up your knees with a blanket roll or two pillows. Although this position seems uncomfortable at first, it often gives prompt relief. Later, you will want to use the same bedding in the flat position for several months or years during recovery.

For the first 24 to 48 hours of treatment, you must stay in bed continuously, use a bed pan as necessary, and eat your meals in bed. Use extreme care never to stretch or stiffen the back. Let your body weight press into the jackknife angle to ease tightness in your back muscles.

2. Learn to keep the lower back flat while carrying on normal activities by taking a series of exercises in bed. Start by lying on your back with your knees bent and your feet flat on the bed. Roll the pelvis forward, as if you were a burlesque artist doing a bump. Hold it for three to five seconds, with the muscles of your abdomen and buttocks tense and hard. Relax for several seconds and repeat 5 to 10 times. Then draw up one knee toward your armpit, pulling with both hands. Draw up the other knee, stretching the back muscles thoroughly. Repeat the whole procedure several times a day. After you have mastered this back-flattening technique of tilting your pelvis, try to keep your pelvis tipped and your lower back flat as you straighten one leg at a time and then as you raise your head and shoulders.

3. Learn to get out of bed, stand, and move about without ever letting a hollow appear in your lower back. Keep one knee clutched against your chest while you are getting your other foot on the ground at first, until you learn to get up without letting your back arch backward. Use the wall as a guide while you learn to stand and move. Stand with your feet four to six inches away from the wall and your back flattened against it. Keep your spine flat against the wall as you raise first one leg, then the other. Squat down and stand back up again without letting your spinal curve change. Keep the spinal curve unchanged as you shift your weight onto your toes and rock away from the wall, then back to it. Finally, walk away from the wall with your lower back completely flat and your pelvis tipped forward instead of back.

4. Learn to perform even extreme bodily movements without letting a

hollow form over your lower spine. Lie on your back with your knees bent and your feet flat on the bed, keep your back flattened and touch your toes with your fingertips. Stand up and keep your back flat as you squat down on your heels and return to the standing position.

5. Drill yourself in assuming all the positions and carrying out all the motions which your job requires without ever letting a hollow form in the small of your back.

This program for curing back injuries works. Take aspirin four times a day after each meal and at bedtime to keep comfortable while you apply rest, exercise, and retraining: two tablets at a dose if you weigh less than 150 pounds, three to a dose if you weigh more. Check Chapter 1 for further measures you can apply for any nagging, persistent back discomfort.

How to prevent recurrent back injuries. Your back ligaments never heal quite as strong as they started. If you once injure your back, you can often save yourself a lot of misery by watching your footing, keeping your back upright while you lift, and by lifting with your legs instead of your back.

When your doctor can give worthwhile aid with backache and back injury. Your doctor can always give worthwhile aid with these three kinds of back trouble:

1. Back pain without strain, injury, or overuse often stems from disease of the kidneys, reproductive organs, spinal column or other vital body parts. Your doctor can identify the source of such trouble, and usually can give quick, permanent relief.

2. Back pain following a severe fall or injury deserves a doctor's care on the spot. If a bone is broken in the spine, there is definite risk of lifelong damage to the spinal cord even if pain is not severe. Your doctor can keep that risk under control.

3. Any back trouble that persists in spite of home measures or requires strong, prescription-only medicines for its relief deserves a doctor's care. In most such cases, your doctor can bring relief with a more intense program based on the same principles outlined above. In a few cases, special braces, injections, or surgery may prove to be the quickest means of getting well.

HOW TO HEAL CUTS, SCRAPES, AND BURNS

You can heal most minor injuries with simple home measures. Four key steps are:

1. Clean the wound.
2. Keep germs from getting in.

3. Improve circulation.
4. Bandage or splint to assure rest and protection as the wound heals.

How to tell when you can get worthwhile help from a doctor for cuts, scrapes or burns. Your doctor can speed healing of most cuts, scrapes, and burns.

A cut that goes all the way through the skin heals more quickly if it is pulled together, either with tape or with stitches. You can tell whether the cut is deep enough to need such care by moving one edge in and out or back and forth. If you can move one edge more than an eighth of an inch without the other edge moving, your doctor can help you with stitches or taping.

Scraped places may have ground-in dirt that you can't scrub loose without undue pain. If so, see your doctor. Be sure your lockjaw protection is up to date if animal wastes may have been tracked into the area where you were injured, or if you cannot wash to the very bottom of the wound.

A burn that turns dead-white or scorched in the center deserves a doctor's care no matter how small it is. Large blistering burns benefit by measures you can't easily apply at home.

Your doctor has tremendous weapons against infection nowadays. Redness, swelling, red streaks up your arm or leg, sore kernels in your neck, armpit or groin, throbbing pain, fever, or chills call for germ-killing medicines, which will work much more quickly if you let your doctor put them to work for you right away.

How to clean out a cut or scrape. The first thing to do for a cut or scrape is to wash with soap and water. Clean your hands thoroughly as you start—hands normally have more germs than any other surface part of your body. Then wash the wound, using either gauze pads or clean, ironed handkerchiefs as washcloths. Soap the cloth and wash with gentle rubbing while the sore is actually in a soft stream of water from a spigot or pitcher. Use at least one quart of water for each wound.

Soap and water actually prevent five times as many infections as any antiseptic used in the depths of a wound. Antiseptics used in a scrape or cut kill tiny portions of the tender tissue underneath your skin. This leaves dead material as food for any remaining germs, and actually does harm instead of good.

How to use antiseptics. The next thing to do is put an antiseptic paint like mercurochrome, merthiolate or metaphen on the normal skin around your sore. Germs always can be found inside the sweat glands, even on freshly washed skin. If you do nothing about these germs, they work back to the surface, rub along the inside of the bandage, and get into your wound within twenty minutes. Antiseptic on the unbroken skin cuts down the number of germs that get into the sore without doing any damage to living tissue. Use antiseptics, but use them *around* a wound instead of *inside* it.

How to improve circulation in the healing sore. Better circulation gives better ability to fight germs and quicker healing. Gentle pressure of an elastic bandage applied smoothly from foot to knee helps leg wounds by keeping down swelling and congestion. Propping an injured leg above breast level also helps. On the hand or arm, you usually need a sling to keep the hurt part up, so that blood runs downhill to the heart. You can rig a sling out of a square yard of muslin or sheet. Fold the square diagonally to make a triangular bandage. Tie the two sharp corners together at the back of the neck with the wrist resting on the middle of the fold and the bandage's blunt angle at the elbow. Adjust so that the lower arm is comfortably raised. Pull the excess cloth back until the sling is smooth from wrist to elbow, fold this excess around the elbow and pin it to the inside surface of the sling.

How to bandage a cut or scrape. The final thing to do for a sore is treat it gently and protect it as it heals. If injured tissue from beneath the skin or healing tissue is exposed, put some petroleum jelly or mild antiseptic ointment on the inside of the bandages or use bandages with plastic lined pads (Telfa) to avoid sticking. If you get hurt on your hands or arms, make your bandage six or eight layers thick to brace the parts and keep them from moving too much. I remember one patient who had a small cut on his finger, for instance.

"I've been fooling with this for a week," he said to me. "It just won't heal."

The cut was shallow and short, but it ran along the side of one finger joint. Whenever he bent his finger, the wound gaped open. His body couldn't build healing tissue fast enough on such shifting ground. A bulky bandage, in this case stiffened with a few matchstick-sized bits of wood, allowed his cut to mend in two days.

Internal zinc. Recent studies have shown that most people in America do not get enough zinc in their diet to achieve maximum wound healing. Cuts, scrapes and even surgical incisions healed one third faster when patients took 80 mcg. of zinc daily. This material is present in some vitamin-mineral capsules like Vi Con C or can be obtained in nutrition shops.

The instant freeze for burns. The most dramatically helpful home measure for burns is undoubtedly the instant freeze. I've seen dozens of injuries which would have gone on to blister formation or worse stopped almost instantly by immediate cold applications. Not only does this program give prompt pain relief, it also cuts down on tissue damage and may prevent weeks of misery.

You need take no precautions against ice burns from overchilling, as described for other forms of cold application. Just get maximum cold to the spot as quickly as possible. Instant application of ice or snow is ideal. If large areas are burned, ice water soaks or compresses may spread the effect to make maximum use of available ice. If ice or snow are not available, perhaps you can get ice-cold water from a drinking fountain, or run the tap water until it is extremely cold. Whatever means you use, try to chill the part as much as possible and keep it chilled for at least fifteen minutes. Pain usually will disappear almost instantly with adequate chilling. Return of pain is a good guide to need for further cold applications. With severe burns, pain may return as soon as the part warms up, and cold applications must be replaced within five or ten minutes. With milder burns, discomfort only gradually reasserts itself, and applications for fifteen minutes every hour for two or three hours suffices. Generally speaking, any burn which requires constant chilling for more than one hour involves enough tissue damage to make a physician's care worthwhile. Danger of shock or other complications makes medical attention necessary with any burn covering more than ten per cent of the body surface.

Immediate chilling helps so much with burns that I would give it priority even over cleanliness. Even if you have to fish the ice out of someone's water glass or scoop up dirty snow from the side of the road, chill that burn instantly! You'll be amazed at the results.

Flame burns. If you burn yourself in a direct flame, the heat usually kills any germs present. Even though the wound looks grimy from soot, you can treat it as being already cleaned. Use the freeze treatment first, of course, then follow up in this way: Reddened areas without change in skin texture respond to greasy ointments like Burn Ointment U.S.P., which you can buy at any drugstore without a prescription. Blistered or scorched areas call for bandaging with petroleum jelly or Telfa. If you are going to see your doctor, cover the burn with a sterile gauze pad or with a freshly ironed handkerchief rather than use grease.

Scalds and other nonflame burns. Wash with soap and water and bandage exactly like a scrape or cut. Several layers of gauze or of fluffed handkerchiefs followed by a snug elastic bandage help to make smooth, even pressure. If blisters become as large as a quarter, you can speed healing by cutting off the dead skin roof. Use manicure scissors which have been flamed or soaked in alcohol, and similarly sterilized tweezers. Keep the scissors blades parallel to the skin and nick the edge of the blister. Insert one scissors blade in the nick and cut around the blister top near its edge, steadying the freed tissue with your tweezers. Discard the blister roof and bandage with petroleum-jelly-coated gauze or Telfa, several gauze pads and a snug gauze or elastic bandage.

Frostbite. Before I moved to Minnesota, the words "biting cold" didn't really mean anything to me. Cold was a penetrating, dank discomfort that went on to make you shiver with chill, not a painful pincer on exposed fingers, nose and ears. Here one almost welcomes painful blasts of wind—frostbite starts with numbness, so you begin to worry when discomfort ends! But cold injury in one form or another can occur anywhere, even in the balmiest climates, and folks all over the world could benefit from experience at Frostbite Falls.

Prevention still helps more than any cure. A lot of cold injury comes from exposure (below freezing) to parts chilled by damp clothing or immersion in slightly too-cold water. I've seen "trench foot" in spring and fall canoe campers who wore wet tennis shoes through a cold snap, for instance. Other cases stem from tight, binding clothes which both carry cold through at the creases and cut down circulation in the part. We've had a rash of frost injury lately due to snow-mobiling in ordinary winter clothes—the extra air movement as you swish around at forty miles an hour can nip an exposed finger or ear in a hurry.

Emergency treatment can make a tremendous difference when numbness, color change or loss of feeling makes you suspect cold injury. Most injury seems to occur through cold-induced spasm of blood vessels rather than tissue freezing itself. Warm soaks or compresses are the best way to open up those blood vessels again. However, if you apply heat directly to the affected part, warmth increases tissue need for fuel even faster than it increases circulation, and can occasionally cause both pain and further damage. You can get full benefit from warm applications by applying the warm compress to the affected body part (arm, leg, etc.) above the site of injury rather than to the injured zone itself. For a frostbitten hand, soak or compress the whole arm from the wrist up rather than from the wrist down, for instance—you'll open the blood vessels in the affected area without increasing tissue oxygen need. The hand itself can be loosely surrounded with flannel or wool to help hold warmth as the increased blood flow brings it, but should not be included in the soak or compress.

There are some body parts where this approach is not practical, of course. You can't soak your head for a frostbitten ear, and frostbite sometimes occurs on the torso where clothing creases or gapes. In these areas, direct thawing works best.

In either case, the water temperature should be 105 degrees, preferably measured with a candy or bath thermometer. Immersing an air thermometer will work, but usually the glass is so thick that temperature readings are not accurate for five minutes or so. If you do not have a thermometer, make the water lukewarm rather than hot—105 is considerably below the top temperature a healthy skin can stand (112 to 120 degrees depending on past dishwashing and similar exposure). *Never thaw a part which might become frozen again* before final treatment—this step makes gangrene and loss of tissue almost inevitable.

One of the absolute worst things for you when you have any form of frostbite is tobacco. Nicotine causes spasm in the blood vessels leading to already-bloodstarved frozen parts. One study showed that almost three times as many frostbite victims had enough gangrene to require amputation of a finger or other body part when they smoked after the injury. Even in milder cases, healing time almost doubled when the patient smoked.

Any frostbite or cold injury which goes on to form blisters or in which sense of touch does not come back deserves a doctor's care. Cold injuries are notorious for seeming mild when later developments prove that they were serious. Above all, don't break blisters or apply any ointment, jelly or poultice—if the injury seems to require these measures, the possibility of lasting damage always justifies professional care.

Splinters. You can remove most splinters for yourself with a flamed needle and a pair of tweezers. Two key points: always unroof a splinter as far as possible before you try to move it, and always tease the splinter loose with the needle point before you try to pick it out with the tweezers. Here's the step-by-step technique:

Clean the area thoroughly with rubbing alcohol. Pass the point of your needle through a flame several times. Slide the tip of the needle a hair's breadth into the hole along the splinter's upper surface. Turn the needle shaft down until it is parallel with the skin and lift up on its point, pulling loose a flake of dead surface skin. Repeat until one eighth of an inch or more of the splinter has been unroofed. Hook the tip of the needle underneath the exposed base of the splinter and gently test to see whether you can lift it. If so, move the splinter up and down and from side to side a couple of times. Transfer the needle to your left hand, and take the tweezers in your right hand. Lift up the splinter end with the point of the needle so that you can grasp it firmly with the tweezers, and remove it. Usually no bandage is necessary.

Splinters under a fingernail. You can cut a wedge of nail off of the top of a splinter and lift it free much more easily than you can pull it out the way it went in. Soak the finger in warm water for twenty minutes to soften the nail. Wipe it off with rubbing alcohol. Use the corner of an alcohol-soaked, clean razor blade. Start over the point of the splinter and make a shallow cut toward the end of the finger along one side of the splinter's shaft. Go back to the point of the splinter, and make another shallow cut toward the end of the finger in such a way that a small pie-shaped wedge of nail is defined over the splinter. Go over these shallow cuts several times, deepening them evenly. You will have to lighten your pressure as you approach the nail margin to keep from cutting yourself as the razor slips off the nail. When the cuts in the nail seem to be nearly or completely through, snip these neglected parts at the margin with scissors and peel the wedge back toward its point. Lift the splinter free with a needle point and pick it out. The wedge defect in the nail will disappear as the nail grows out.

Gouged out wounds. If you tear or cut out a bit of skin, the resulting wound is often quite painful. Small gouges will heal up with simple home measures, though. Put an old, freshly ironed handkerchief in a small covered oven dish with about an ounce of petroleum jelly. Heat in the oven until the petroleum jelly melts and soaks in the cloth. Let cool. Cut a piece of this material large enough to fold into three or four layers over the wound. Cover with a gauze and adhesive bandage. Change the bandage once a day. If the wound heals normally, pinkish proud flesh will form in two or three days, then grayish skin cells will make a pearly, glistening margin that gradually closes the defect. If the proud flesh heaps up so that the skin cells have to grow uphill, let your doctor burn them down with special chemicals. As soon as the whole wound has grayish, glistening tissue across it, you can omit further bandaging. A little cold cream rubbed into the area once or twice a day helps to keep the tender healing tissue from cracking open again.

CHOKING

A few conditions are certainly serious enough to warrant a doctor's care, but are so urgent that you usually have to depend on home measures simply because the doctor could not get there on time. You'll find good guidance for most of these, such as bleeding, drowning and shock, in first aid books from the Red Cross or the Boy Scouts of America, which you probably have lying around the house. But most of those books (unless they're brand new) don't contain much material on choking. The Heimlich maneuver, which saves many of the people who would die before an ambulance could come, has only been in use for a few short years, and hasn't worked its way into many first aid manuals.

When someone chokes on a piece of food or the like, the foreign material blocks flow of air through the voice box, so the victim cannot holler for help or tell you what is wrong. His violent efforts to get air into his lungs look like some kind of sudden spasm, and he quickly loses consciousness and falls out of his chair. Dr. Heimlich has advised a "universal sign" of choking—a sort of manual SOS—in which the victim puts both hands up to his throat. If you and your loved ones learn that gesture, it may some day save one of your lives. But I wouldn't depend on it entirely: always check for choking whenever a sudden spasm or abrupt unconsciousness strikes, especially at the table or at a party. Peanuts and chewing gum, alcohol (which dulls the reflexes with which your body protects itself against choking), and sudden laughter (which sometimes sucks food into the voice box) are often factors.

When a person chokes, air flow through his nose and mouth do not occur. Lack of air flow, as detected with a wisp of tissue where the airstream should be, while the victim is making violent efforts to breathe, shows that he has choked.

In this situation, your treatment aims at producing a sudden rush of air up through the windpipe to dislodge the blocking bit of food. You cannot do this by squeezing on the chest, because the ribs won't move inward quickly enough. But you can push abdominal organs upward against the diaphragm, which in turn will push upward against the lungs. Get behind the victim and reach around with both hands. Clasp your hands together in such a way that the knuckle at the base of your thumb pushes into the pit of his stomach. Give a sharp upward and inward squeeze, hopefully popping the food particle loose like the cork in a champagne bottle.

In the rare case where the victim is an infant or small child, you can produce the same effect by placing him on a flat surface and pressing inward and upward on the pit of his stomach with both thumbs.

Sometimes this maneuver doesn't work the first time because of muscular spasm holding the piece of food in place. When the victim passes out, the spasm usually relaxes. So try again and again if the situation seems to be getting worse or continuing. The worse off the victim is, the better the chance that the maneuver will work.

14

Tonics and Correctives That Build Your Strength and Energy

As you drive through northern Minnesota, you will often notice a small windowless concrete hut nestled close to the shore of some river or lake. Don't make the mistake of calling the blond giants in the vicinity Swedes! They're almost certainly Finnish in descent, and quite proud of it. The concrete huts prove their dedication to a tone-up ritual originating in the Old Country, and unexcelled anywhere in the world—the famous "sauna." By pouring water on hot rocks, participants fill the little huts with thick, hot steam. The novices lie near the floor, while old hands rest on shelves closer to the ceiling where the rising heat may reach 140° F. The thick, moist warmth increases circulation in their naked skin until it looks quite flushed. Brisk flailing with wooden switches brings still more blood to the surface, whereupon the order of the day becomes a plunge in icy water. Surprisingly, the cold fluid feels like warm syrup to the still hot hide. When it begins to chill, a brisk toweling and warm clothes are close at hand. If you want a new sensation of vigor and vitality, any Finn will tell you that a sauna never fails!

We'll say more about home saunas later in this chapter, but most people must resort to less vigorous tonic methods for lack of equipment, companions, or courage. If you find weariness draining away the pleasures of life and keeping you from doing your best, if you find modern racecourse living imposing intolerable burdens of nervous and physical fatigue, if you suffer fatigue-inducing disorders or distress—you can certainly benefit from tonic techniques that build strength, zest, and energy. The tried-and-true methods described in this chapter help to combat everyday weariness and irritability, improve your mood and resistance, and nullify conditions that drag you down. Detailed directions will help you to fight five common disorders which increase fatigue, and to get effective help for several others.

HOW TO FIGHT TENSION AND FATIGUE WITH
LIFE'S GREAT NATURAL TONICS

Perfectly normal, healthy people often need a soothing, reviving tonic technique. Tension builds up, irritability and restlessness cause distress, and blue moods or living reverses take their toll. Even for everyday vicissitudes, home tonic procedures are worthwhile. For paralyzing tension or depression, they help even more.

Part-by-part relaxation. The most important single way to conserve your energy is to dissolve excess tension with deliberate relaxation. When you are tense, every muscle in your body is working. You use just as much physical energy as if you were walking continuously at a rapid clip. No wonder you feel exhausted by the end of the day!

You can control tension and intensify the benefits of rest through the technique of part-by-part relaxation. Ordinary rest or simple relaxation leaves muscles in their basic state of tension. Deliberate, part-by-part relaxation goes beyond this point to deliberately probed depths of laxity. Here is the basic method:

> Lie on your back in a quiet room with your arms at your sides and your legs uncrossed. Deliberately relax your scalp muscles, your face muscles, then your neck. (If you have difficulty getting the muscles to relax at first, learn to relax by exaggerating muscle stiffness, then eliminating it. Hold your neck stiffer and stiffer by stages until it is extremely stiff. Then hold it not quite so stiff, still looser, and looser still. When you get back to normal tension, continue the same process by which you have moved from stiff to normal, and move on from normal to relaxed.) When your scalp, face, and neck seem fairly relaxed, move on to other parts of the body. Relax your right arm and hand, then your right leg, left leg, and left arm. Next, stretch your breathing muscles. Slowly take a deep breath through your nose, inflating your lungs as far as possible with your diaphragm, then further with the chest muscles. Let the breath escape gently through your mouth. Repeat the breathing exercise three times. Start with the scalp again, and impose even more complete relaxation on each of your body parts.

Part-by-part relaxation is fundamental to tonic techniques. The most universally applicable, and easiest to learn, is the *rest break with part-by-part relaxation*. A rest break during the day with part-by-part relaxation is three to six times as effective as the same amount of extra rest at night. Most workers find the twenty minutes or half hour before supper an ideal time for a rest break, while housewives more commonly take their time off after lunch. The room should be darkened and quiet if possible. If physical weariness plagues you, extra benefit stems from propping your legs and arms on pillows. The knees should be slightly bent with the lower legs parallel to the floor on two pillows each. Turn your hands palm down on one pillow each with your arms slightly out from your sides. A very small pillow or rolled towel under the neck usually works better than a big, soft pillow. Follow the basic method for part-by-part relaxation described above.

Rest periods can do a great deal for you, as Herman Saunders found out shortly after he was promoted to service manager at a large automobile agency.

"I'm racking myself up at work," he told me. "Between being on my feet all the time and constant pressure, I'm so tired and tense that I'm not worth a hang by afternoon."

There was nothing wrong with Herman except the natural effects of new responsibility and a heavy work load. A noon hour rest break helped a lot. He took a full hour lunch period, ate in twenty minutes, and followed the relaxation routine you've just read about for half an hour before he started back for work.

Result? Two years later, Herman won a trip to Canada for running the best service department in his district.

"Thanks to that noon-hour-break," he told me, "I can keep a smile on my face and some starch in my back all through the day, and still find the energy someplace for a little social life."

Insomnia-combatting relaxation. Once you have learned to relax in the face of normal tension you can apply the same technique against stresses and worries which are robbing you of sleep. In a sense, loss of sleep is less of a problem than *concern* about loss of sleep. You toss around in bed frantically repeating to yourself:

"I've got to go to sleep! I won't be worth a hang tomorrow if I don't get to sleep!"

You not only lose sleep, you get absolutely no rest!

If you put part-by-part relaxation to work for you, all this is changed. Actual measurement has shown that energy expenditure declines farther with part-by-part relaxation than with sleep—proof that resting time used in this way is actually more efficient than sleep itself. You don't have to roll and toss and worry about whether you'll be any good in the morning: relax and restore your full capacities, whether you sleep or not! Just follow the basic method described above with one exception: if you find it difficult to relax a whole arm or a whole leg in the face of worry and strain, break down the area to smaller and smaller parts. Relax your hand, your forearm and your upper arm, or even one finger at a time, instead of your whole arm at once.

You can use this technique even if you've always thought of yourself as a born, incurable worry-wart. One of my patients, Peter Sanford, didn't believe that he would ever banish the worry whirl from his sleepless brain.

"I've used sleeping pills for years," he told me. "Whenever I get into a financial hole or have a family argument—anything upsetting—I need medicine to put me to sleep. No matter how I try to control my thoughts, the same old worries and tensions keep popping into my mind."

"Just try this method," I told him. "I'm sure you'll be able to master it."

A few months later, Peter Sanford was back in my office.

"I haven't taken a single sleeping pill for five months," he told me. "That relaxation technique really works! Took me a few weeks to get the hang of it, but I've felt great ever since. Funny thing, when you don't fight to get to sleep, you usually forget your worries and drop off in a hurry, too."

More serious forms of insomnia. Relaxation doesn't help everyone with disturbed sleep. There are two forms you can recognize at home, but which call for prompt medical treatment.

The first is *sleep apnea*. Victims of this disorder generally complain of being tired all the time and falling to sleep at inappropriate times. One of my recent patients told me: "I fall asleep right in the middle of a conversation with a customer." Another had an automobile accident from falling asleep at the wheel. If this condition stems from sleep apnea, relatives usually mention that the victim snores very loudly, and sometimes that he or she thrashes around a lot in the bed.

Victims of sleep apnea simply relax so thoroughly when they sleep that the walls of their air passages collapse. This blocks breathing, and they struggle for air, often by thrashing around and gasping loudly until they become sufficiently awake to open up the air passages. This problem originally came to light in fat, middle-aged men, but the more we learn about it the more we recognize that the fatness comes from being inactive (from being worn out all the time). Several of the patients whom I have found suffering from this disorder have been slim, and one was only twelve years old. The tip-off—the thing you can easily spot right at home—is periods of blocked breathing during sleep. Usually if you sit up and watch the victim as he sleeps, you will note frequent periods when he simply quits breathing for half a minute or more, followed by restlessness and gasping for breath. In some cases it helps to tape a small wisp of Kleenex to the victim's nose so that you can tell when no air is moving in and out through his nose.

If nothing is done about sleep apnea, serious aftereffects may develop. The breathless periods cause lack of oxygen in the brain and the heart, and some patients even die from the resulting damage. If you have any reason to suspect this condition, any well-informed doctor can arrange permanent and very effective care.

The other dangerous form of insomnia stems from *depression*. This form of disturbed sleep differs from ordinary insomnia in that the victim usually goes to sleep without much trouble, then wakes very early and tosses and turns for hours before wake-up time arrives. Most victims of depression also complain of fatigue and difficulty getting started in the morning. Some note blue moods, crying when alone, lack of appetite, fall-off in sex drive, and constipation. If any two of these complaints are present in addition to disturbed sleep, a doctor's care almost always proves worthwhile.

The tension-easing refresher slouch. When you have mastered bed-bound relaxation in the face of stresses and worry, you can apply the technique in the upright position to keep tension from building up in the first place. Used in this way, a tension-easing break works wonders for your temperament and your efficiency. Best technique: the refresher slouch.

> Sit in a straight chair with both feet flat on the floor. Let your hands rest relaxed in your lap, with your shoulders sagging forward. Close your eyes and let your head hang loose in front of your chest. Relax as completely as possible, part by part. Continue deliberate relaxation until you cannot feel stiffness or tension anywhere in your body. This usually takes about one minute. Then lift your right hand to shoulder height and let it fall limply into your lap again. Do the same with your left hand. Try to relax part by part even more completely. After another minute, you will find that you are able to take up the cares of the day in a much more relaxed and comfortable way.

How often should you use the tension-breaking refresher slouch? That depends on how much pressure you must withstand. Every housewife should work a refresher slouch into her schedule during the hectic pre-supper hour. Most businessmen need a midmorning and midafternoon break. Some of my patients average almost one break an hour, which still involves no real lost time: they find boosted efficiency and mental calm makes many brief rest breaks worthwhile. Check your own day for tension-ridden hours, and interrupt such periods with two minute breaks. You'll find them very helpful.

Tranquilizing tubs. Next to part-by-part relaxation, the most readily available home remedy for fatiguing irritability and jangled nerves is the tranquilizing tub. This tonic technique works especially well when things are getting you down—when you feel blue and depressed, and life hardly seems worth living. It also helps built-up tension and insomnia. All you need is a bathtub, two towels, some string and a floating or candy-making thermometer to get considerable relief. Here's how to do it:

Fill your tub with water at 94 to 98 degrees Fahrenheit. Roll one towel so that it forms a tube with the upper end around the faucet and the lower end trailing in the water. Attach it to the faucet with string or with a strong rubber band. This will act as a wick and keep the flow of water into the tub silent—otherwise the constant dribbling noise is annoying. Be sure the overflow drain in the tub works properly. Get into the tub. Turn the water back on, adjusting to a slow flow of lukewarm water. The water flowing into the tub usually has to be kept at about 100 degrees in order to overcome cooling by evaporation and to keep the tub continuously at 94 to 98 degrees. A little experience will soon show what flow and what temperature work the best.

When the tub is adjusted, arrange the second towel in a small pillow-like roll and place it behind your neck to support your head as you lie back in relaxed comfort. Stay in the tub for at least a half hour. The soothing effect increases with duration. Many patients find baths up to two or three hours worthwhile, especially when they have been very upset or blue.

Tranquilizing tub treatments can help pull you out of the very depths of gloom. They can also help you shuck off the cares and worries of daily life. Try them: you'll be surprised at how effective they can be.

Wet sheet packs. Wet sheet packs are less easily managed than other home measures against wearying tension or depression because you must induce a member of your family to learn and apply this method before you can enjoy its benefits. The technique is much easier than it sounds, though: after you have gone through the routine once or twice, you will find that you can get into a pack in two minutes or less. The soothing effect helps anyone who has been under extra pressure, and is powerful enough to calm victims of even extreme external or internal strain. If you feel the need for inner peace or uplift, whether from normal living strains or from some severe disturbance, try a wet sheet pack. The only special equipment required is a sheet of plastic, rubber, or oilcloth. You will also use two wool blankets, an ordinary bed sheet, a basin or tub, and your bed. Here's the step by step technique:

Spread a wool blanket on the bed, then a sheet of plastic, rubber, or oilcloth on top. Partly fill a basin with cold water, between 60 and 70 degrees

Fahrenheit. Undress and lie on your side at the edge of the bed away from your helper, facing away from him. Have your helper dip the folded sheet in the cold water and wet it thoroughly. Then have him wring it out and spread it quickly along the middle of the bed, the top about one inch from the top of the blanket and the side toward you gathered into lengthwise pleats which will spread easily. Now roll onto the cold, wet sheet. You may shiver for a few moments, but the discomfort will pass quickly. Have your helper spread the sheet completely. Raise your arms above your head. Have your helper wrap one half of the sheet around your body, with its top end high under the armpits. Lower your arms. Have your helper wrap the other half of the sheet around your arms and all, with its upper border diagonal across your chest and its upper corner under the back of your neck. Now have your helper press the sheet down between your legs and fold the end loosely underneath your feet. The sheet should be snug, but not tight.

Next your helper should fold one half of the blanket and its waterproof covering across your body and tuck it in, then the other half. By this time you should be feeling warm and relaxed. Another blanket or two, a pillow or folded towel under your neck, a well-padded hot water bottle near your feet if necessary, and you will enjoy from thirty to sixty minutes of wonderfully complete calm.

One caution: wet sheet packs work well only when they are applied rapidly. It's a good idea to go through a dry run or two with your helper before you wet the sheet: otherwise you will get into your pack so slowly that you will be chilled instead of warmed and relaxed by it.

Soothing massage. Massage is the least available of the great natural tonics because it takes so much practiced assistance. If you are lucky enough to have someone who is willing to learn how to give massage and spend half to three-quarters of an hour giving you each treatment, it is often very soothing. Here's the technique:

Wear loose, easily adjusted clothing such as a nightgown or a pair of shorts. Lie down in a comfortable position, with extra pillows if you need them. Uncover one arm, and have your helper powder it thoroughly with talc. Let your muscles go completely loose: don't try to help in any way. Now your helper should begin slowly and gently stroking the exposed arm, working from the shoulder down. His movements should be perfectly rhythmic, with his hand traveling in a steady oval: down the arm, lift and up again, down the arm, and so on. He should use his other hand to support the arm and to change its position. It is important that the strokes be always in the same direction, and that the massaging hand be gently applied and gently lifted so that there is no sense of jarring at the beginning or end. Your helper's nails should never scratch your skin at the end of a stroke.

The stroking should increase gradually in frequency and vigor as your helper moves along from shoulder to hand, then to the other arm and to the legs. When all the extremities have been massaged, you should turn over. Similar stroking of the neck and back, this time with both hands at once, makes a good conclusion to massage. The movements should taper to gentle, slow ones as the massage is ended.

Lethargy-fighting tonics. Although tension causes more fatigue than any other factor in American life, some people manage to slough it off without difficulty. In fact, the main complaint many of my patients express is difficulty getting started.

"Nothing bothers me," one of them told me the other day. "In fact, nothing seems to matter much at all. I've felt sometimes that there was something missing—some inner drive or interest or ambition or something—that would really help me make something of my life. But that's just the way I'm built, I guess."

This patient got a tremendous lift out of the next of life's great natural tonics: the *cold friction bath*. Check with your doctor before taking cold friction baths if you have high blood pressure, heart disease, or extreme nervous irritability. Don't take cold baths if you are highly subject to chilblains or to hives brought on by cold exposure. Otherwise, give them a try if you can't get cracking: you'll probably find that cold friction baths make you feel 20 years younger for several hours at a time, and fill you with extra energy and zest. They also often improve your circulation and increase resistance to head colds. The technique is simple and takes little time.

Bundle up well and drink a cup of warm cocoa while you fill your tub. Adjust the temperature of the water to between seventy and eighty degrees Fahrenheit. Undress and get into the bath quickly, immersing your whole body up to the chin. You will gasp for breath for a few moments, but that discomfort will soon pass. If possible, have someone in your family rub the entire surface of your body briskly with both hands all the while you are under the water. Otherwise rub all parts of your own body vigorously yourself with both hands. If the rubbing is sufficiently vigorous, you will feel comfortably warm for from one-half minute to three minutes. Get out of the bath the moment you start to feel chilly. As soon as you get out of the bath, rub yourself briskly with a coarse towel. When as dry as possible, switch to another coarse, dry towel and rub briskly for another two minutes.

Cold friction baths can be made gradually colder and longer as you become accustomed to them. Take them at least twice a week for maximum effect. Lower the temperature about two degrees each time. You will find that you can become accustomed to temperatures down into the fifties if rubbing is sufficiently vigorous.

Home saunas. Anyone who has sweated his way through a home sauna will think I am crazy for saying so, but the main effect comes from *cold* application, not from *hot*. All the ritual of working up a giant sweat simply makes a cold dip or shower comfortable enough to endure. In fact, once the blood is racing through your overheated skin, a cold dip or shower feels more like warm honey than ice water, and (except for a bit of initial gasping when each body area is exposed to a new level of cold) you almost never feel chilled with the coldest water flow you can get through your bathroom's pipes.

You have to be able to stand all that stimulation before a sauna is any good to you, and the same limitations cited above for cold friction baths (blood pressure, heart disease, nervous irritability, chilblains, cold-related hives) apply here. There's also very real danger of giddiness or fainting from standing up too quickly while your body is overheated. Warmth opens up all your body's blood vessels, and sudden change of posture can let blood detour to the legs in such quantity that your brain gets no circulation. Best change from lying to sitting to standing only with a considerable pause between stages until your body builds tolerance to heat.

If you observe these limitations, a home sauna can be a great pick-me-up. Never take a sauna when you have been out in the cold during the last two hours—even brief, mild cold exposure ruins your skin's responsiveness. Sip a little salted broth or Gatorade (or similar product) to avoid heat exhaustion effects, and use a cold towel around the neck if necessary to avoid headache. Sit in the heat until you are sweating all over your body, including your palms and the soles of your feet, which usually takes about twenty minutes—twice as long as it takes to make your face sweat heavily. Move promptly to either a shower or tub for the cold bath part of the program.

If a shower, start with lukewarm water and turn it gradually colder, rubbing with your hands in the area where the water hits and turning to get each part of your body accustomed to every temperature change. You will gasp slightly for breath as the water gets colder, but this will quickly pass. If you get a good blood-vessel reaction, you will feel as if your head is suddenly becoming super-clear. This feeling will usually increase for a minute or two after the bath gets really cold, then reach a stationary plane. At that point, before you begin to feel chilled, get out of the shower and dry yourself briskly, using a second dry towel for a thirty-second rubdown at the end.

If you must use a tub, fill the tub with the coldest water available before your sauna (because you won't have time to fill it afterward). By the time you are ready to use it, the water will have warmed slightly. Follow the procedure described above for cold friction baths, which you will find comfortable with much colder water after working up a good sweat "hot rocks" style.

How to tone up flabby muscles and do-nothing nerves with a sheet bath. If someone in your family will help you, here's a way to tone yourself up with very little mess or bother. You can enjoy the stimulation of a sheet bath with very little equipment or space. Here's how to do it:

> Warm one sheet in your oven beforehand, and put it in the bathroom. Gather another sheet from the ends like a drawn curtain. Soak it in water between 60 and 80 degrees Fahrenheit. Take off your clothes and stand in the bathtub or shower stall, preferably with a rubber bath mat to assure good footing. Have your helper hold up the wet sheet. Raise your arms. Have your helper place an upper corner of the wet sheet in your right armpit. Lower your right arm to hold the sheet in place. Turn to your right, wrapping the sheet around under your left arm and across your back. Drop your other arm and turn until your body is completely enveloped in the sheet. Have your helper tuck in the loose upper corner snugly or pin it to hold the sheet in place. Now your helper should immediately rub your body through the sheet, using long, vigorous strokes down the length of your arms, body, and legs. When your helper feels definite surface warmth through the sheet all over your body, he should unwrap you and put on the dry, warm sheet in exactly the same way. Have him continue rubbing with long, vigorous, lengthwise strokes until you are thoroughly dried.

From the beginning to end, a sheet bath takes four to six minutes. Counting preparation time and clean-up, you'll spend less than ten minutes for a new sensation of tingling liveliness. Try it soon!

Sex as a tonic. In a sense, sex is a fair-weather friend. When things are going well for you and your marriage relations are completely cordial, sex adds boundlessly to your energy, tranquility, and contentment. When you are upset or depressed, or when your marriage is going sour, both your sexual capacities and sexual enjoyment suffer severely. You must often use other natural tonics or even medical measures to get yourself in shape for sex, but once you are ready for relaxed indulgence, you'll reap both soothing and stimulating effects.

Don't let temporary sexual impairments add to your worries or depression. A great many of my patients have encountered this vicious circle: tension or depression upsets their sex life, concern about the disturbed sex life leads to further tension or depression, which upsets sex life further still. These unfortunate people often cannot get their lives back on an even keel until they realize that their sexual capacities are not permanently or seriously impaired. For instance, Bill Farnham complained that he could not maintain an erection.

"I'm only forty-five," he told me despondently. "But I must be in my eighties from the waist down."

Bill's troubles had started a few months before, when his daughter eloped with a young man of whom the Farnhams disapproved. During the period of tension that followed, Bill found himself sexually incapable. He became thoroughly alarmed. Every time he developed designs on his loving wife, he spent the whole evening worrying. "Will I be able to make a go of it tonight?" No wonder he was too keyed up for sexual success by the time he got ready for bed!

Like most similar sufferers, Bill Farnham regained his capacities almost overnight as soon as he understood the source of his difficulties. Sexual relations call for a complex fusion of physical and emotional factors, that almost any severely upsetting experience can temporarily upset. If you realize that fact, you will not let an occasional failure under duress add further burdens of doubt and fear. You will avoid vicious-circle type sex incapacity.

Tone up for sex when you suffer depression or jitters. The other great natural tonics we have discussed in this chapter do wonders in preparation for sex. There is no better way to start an evening which will culminate in marital communion than with sheet baths or massage. Sex caps the climax of the other tone-up processes. It is the crowning tonic, to be used only after you have soothed or stimulated yourself out of any accumulated tension or the blues.

HOME CORRECTIVES FOR SEVERAL FREQUENT FATIGUING DISORDERS

One of the worst features of fatigue-causing disorders is that people often suffer with them for years before seeking relief. These problems arise so gradually that victims often think of their low energy store as part of their time of life or as a perfectly normal result of wear and tear. Yet many of these disorders yield quickly to home correctives, and others vanish after inexpensive and painless varieties of prescription care. If you tire more quickly than you think you should, you may find the key to renewed energy and zestful productivity in the next few pages.

How to conquer ordinary low-grade anemia. If the oxygen-carrying strength of your blood is not quite up to its ideal level, you will get a big boost from extra *iron-containing foods*. You should suspect this condition if you tire easily and if your fingernail beds are somewhat paler than those of heartier friends.

Eggs build up your blood. They work especially well if you take them at the same meal with citrus fruits, which help you to digest and make use of egg iron even though they contain little iron themselves. Two eggs with a glass of orange juice should be part of your standard blood-building breakfast.

Meat is another blood builder. A good serving of meat at lunch and at dinner helps fight off borderline anemia. You can use organ meats like liver, heart, and kidneys to keep down the cost if you wish: they are just as effective as expensive steaks and chops.

Iron tablets. Iron pills are also cheap and safe. The best form of iron pills for low grade anemia is ferrous gluconate. It is both cheaper and better than most blood building tonic mixtures. Since iron soaks into your system much more thoroughly when you take it on an empty stomach, you should take three tablets each day, one before each meal. If you are the one person in fifty who gets some heartburn or loss of appetite from ferrous gluconate tablets on this schedule, take them immediately after meals instead. This almost always controls their slight indigestion-spurring effect.

Any form of iron pill may cause your bowel movements to turn black, so don't be alarmed at this change. Some people find iron tablets somewhat constipating: try extra fruit and fluid intake if your pills cause bowel trouble.

Overweight. If you can pinch up a roll of abdominal fat between your thumb and forefinger which is more than one inch thick, you will probably gain substantial extra stores of strength and endurance by losing weight. Chapter 18 details two helpful methods.

Underweight. Underweight people often complain of fatigue, especially late in the morning, afternoon, and evening. The problem here is mainly a lack of fuel reserves. When the calories from your last meal have been exhausted, your muscles and brain have no ready supply of nourishment. You feel dull, depressed, and exhausted. Either ready fuel supply at the time or the fuel reserves of a few extra pounds will give you tremendous help.

Energizing snacks. If you are underweight, or even if you suffer a late morning and afternoon let-down in spite of normal weight, extra energizing snacks are quite worthwhile. Such snacks produce an actual, measured gain in efficiency of 9.7 per cent. An apple, an orange, a bowl of soup or some milk work just as well as the traditional doughnuts and coffee, and offer extra strength-boosting nutritional values.

The lactose weight-gain program. A quickly digested, high sugar snack at the right time will actually increase your appetite for the next meal, thus adding extra mealtime calories as well as its own fuel values to your weight-increasing food supply. When you eat sugar-producing, quickly digested foods, the amount of sugar in your blood increases. Your body uses some of that sugar for quick energy, and lays up more in storage. When the amount of sugar in your blood falls to normal again, your body gradually stops laying up stored supplies. But it can't stop instantly, so your blood sugar level falls well below normal. As long as your blood sugar is below normal, you feel distinctly hungry. This happens for about thirty minutes a little more than an hour after your high-sugar snack or meal.

You need to skip all other between-meals eating, start your meals with the main course, and take rather large amounts of quickly digested carbo-hydrate to produce substantial weight gain. Four heaping tablespoonfuls of sugar is the average effective dose. However, many patients find that amount of plain sugar unbearably sweet and use milk sugar instead. Milk sugar, sold in any drugstore under the chemical name "lactose," gives the same appetite-boosting effect as ordinary sugar, but it is only one-eighth as sweet. Lactose which is pure enough for food use (you don't need expen-sive chemically pure or technical grade) is fairly cheap. You'll find it pleasant to take, too: just stir four heaping tablespoonfuls into tart fruit juice, lemonade, or plain water. Timed exactly one and a half hours before lunch and supper, this dose puts ten pounds onto the average patient in less than a month.

Fatigue from testicular congestion. You can cure fatigue from testicu-lar congestion with very simple home measures. If you have an extra tangle of veins just above the left testicle as big as a walnut or larger, you may be suffering fatigue from testicular congestion. If so, extra scrotal support will definitely increase your strength and energy.

Suspensory. A comfortable elastic scrotal support or suspensory re-lieves testicular congestion at a cost of two dollars or so. Wear a suspensory for a couple of weeks. If it makes you more energetic and less easily fatigued, buy several suspensories and wear one all the time. Otherwise, put your suspensory in the bureau drawer and try again in a year or so: this form of fatigue is so gradual in onset that often the only way you know it is there is by the relief you get from suspensory support.

Fatigue from sexual over-indulgence. An overdose of any tranquilizer leads to torpor, albeit blissful torpor. Sex is no exception. Despite old wives' tales which blame sex-weariness on diet, the plain fact seems to be that it is due to an imbalance in your sympathetic nervous system with over-action of the anti-excitement, anti-stimulation element.

Alternate hot-cold showers. You can often bring the elements of your sympathetic nervous system back into balance after sexual over-indulgence with alternate hot-cold showers. Start with fairly hot water, spraying every part of your body surface. Rub vigorously with both hands in the area being sprayed. Adjust the water to as much heat as you can stand, then abruptly switch to a cold spray. Continue vigorous rubbing until gasping subsides, turning to expose all body parts. The cold spray will then feel comfortable for twenty to thirty seconds. Before you start to feel chilled, switch back to hot water for two minutes or so. Continue alternating hot and cold for about ten minutes, then rub yourself briskly all over with a succession of dry, coarse towels.

Types of fatigue for which your doctor's help is worthwhile. Severe fatigue certainly deserves medical care just as much as disabling pain or other miseries. However, even mild fatigue may point to conditions for which prompt medical care will prove worthwhile. If you know what accompanying signs to watch out for, you will detect the underlying cause of your fatigue sooner and win relief much more quickly than if you wait until severe difficulty drives you to your doctor's office.

Blood loss anemia. If you can stop the loss of a few drops of blood each day, you relieve your blood-forming organs of a great strain. The blood loss may not be alarming—I've had patients who didn't think it was even worth mentioning. But you often gain stronger blood and extra energy by stopping any form of persistent bleeding.

Here are several types of continual bleeding which you may be able to spot, and which your doctor can usually stop with inexpensive and painless measures:

1. Heavy or long-lasting menstrual flow. Periods should last no more than seven days, and should soil about one dozen pads per month. Heavier flow or passage of frequent or large clots deserves medical correction.
2. Bleeding with stools, even if it obviously comes from hemorrhoids.
3. One or more black, bulky stools, especially if they occur after a sudden weak spell. Bleeding into the stomach or intestine often shows up this way because the blood turns black during digestion.
4. Vomiting of bloody or coffee-grounds-like material. Stomach acids change blood into brownish flakes.
5. Frequent or severe nosebleeds.
6. Reddish or blood-tinged urine.

Pernicious anemia. Pernicious anemia resists iron treatment or diet completely, but gets well very promptly with liver or vitamin B_{12} shots. Liver shots might be of tremendous help to you if weakness and tiredness come along with dizzy spells, easy loss of wind, and numbness or tingling of the legs. A tendency to stumble in the dark or to bark your shins frequently also points toward this ailment.

How to conquer fatigue due to a sluggish thyroid. Thyroid hormone makes sluggish body processes speed up. It bestirs energy, keeps your skin and hair healthy, and helps you toward comfortable warmth. Hundreds of thousands of women and tens of thousands of men have found boundless energy in a few cents' worth of thyroid pills a month. These happy people completely, comfortably, and inexpensively replace the thyroid gland products which their own body fails to supply. If you have signs of thyroid deficiency, thyroid pills may offer a safe, inexpensive, and comfortable road to a newly energized life.

When should you suspect thyroid deficiency? If you have three or more of these signs:

1. Dry skin.
2. Coarse or thinning hair.
3. Easy fatigue.
4. Unusual menstruation, either scanty, irregular, heavy, or frequent.
5. Continuous puffiness of eyelids and cheeks (usually so gradual in onset that victims only notice it when they compare their present appearance with old snapshots).
6. Irritability.
7. Sleepiness or sluggishness.
8. Easy chilling—victims often want the room much warmer than other people, and need extra sweaters and extra covers.

Lila Grant found boundless energy and new calm and contentment through thyroid pills. Tension crackled between Lila Grant and her husband, Bill, when they first came to my office.

"For the last three or four years," Bill said, "Lila's been getting worse and worse. She's so irritable it's driving all of us nuts. There must be *something* wrong—she wasn't that way before."

Lila's face was pinched under coarse, dull hair. Her dry-skinned, rough hands were in tight fists.

"I don't know," she said. "Maybe there is something wrong. I fly off the handle over nothing, and I know I shouldn't. But what can I do?"

Tests showed that Lila needed thyroid pills. A few months later, Bill came to my office with her again.

"Lila's got her disposition back again, doctor," he said. "It's simply wonderful what those pills do for her."

That's what most patients say, and their families, too. Whether thyroid lack causes sluggishness or irritability or both, it always causes misery. A few visits to a doctor do a world of good.

How to conquer fatigue from overactive thyroid. An overactive thyroid can be tamed with medicines or surgically removed. Left alone, it makes body processes race at an inefficient rate. If you have an overactive thyroid, your heart races and pounds. You sweat a great deal and feel uncomfortably warm. You lose weight in spite of good appetite. You become nervous and irritable.

An overactive thyroid is usually swollen. You can see definite fullness or a lump a couple of inches down from your Adam's apple. The fullness moves up and down with the Adam's apple when you swallow.

Your doctor can give worthwhile help if you have an overactive thyroid. See him soon if you suspect that this is troubling you.

How to avoid diabetes. Some people can avoid diabetes entirely by discovering and correcting their tendency toward the disease. If you are more than twenty pounds overweight, or if your family background includes many victims of diabetes or of overweight, special tests for diabetic tendencies may be worthwhile. Here's a case which shows what you might accomplish:

When Doris Maxwell was 43, her younger sister developed diabetes. Doris decided she should have a thorough checkup herself, since her mother and brother also suffered the same disease.

Doris did not have diabetes, but her tests showed an abnormal blood-sugar curve. This meant that she was fated for that disease soon, unless she took steps to avoid it. Doris immediately began to eat more meat and eggs and less sugars and starches. Her special diet is not at all hard to follow—no measured quantities or rigid menus. She uses low-calorie substitues for sugar wherever possible and omits excess sweets and starches. For very little money or inconvenience she has kept herself entirely free of diabetes. In fact, she now has a completely normal blood-sugar curve, and is one stage further away from disease than she was five years ago.

How to hold diabetes in check. Even if you do not avoid diabetes altogether, you can probably avoid its ravages. Your doctor can help you to live out virtually your full lifespan in comfort and efficiency. He can keep you from suffering the complaints which victims of uncontrolled diabetes endure. He can slow down the rapid aging to which diabetics are prone.

Every day that diabetes remains unchecked, its victim ages several days to a week. What a terrible waste, when a few cents' worth of medicine a day could stop unduly rapid deterioration! If you fall victim to diabetes, you can keep vigor and strength for many extra years by finding and caring for your disorder promptly.

How can you find it promptly? Most patients complain mainly of fatigue and frequent infections like colds, boils and festering sores. Many lose weight in spite of a good appetite, or eat vast amounts without weight gain. Constant thirst is a tip-off, along with increased urination. But many victims of diabetes never realize that anything serious is wrong until a urine test shows extra sugar. If you're in that group, you could profit tremendously from one new development: home urine-testing kits are now distributed free at drug stores almost everywhere during Diabetes Detection Week (the third week in November). Or you can buy test materials and directions for a few cents per test and check a sample voided about two hours after your main meal. A positive test does not always mean diabetes, but it does mean that you should get your doctor to do further examinations. If you find diabetes early, you'll often restore energy you've forgotten you ever had, and at the same time add many years to your life.

15

How to Improve Your Circulation with Home Measures

When my patients start to talk yearningly of retirement to Florida or California, I can usually bet that they suffer substantial circulatory miseries. While Minnesotans grouse about six months of winter, few would trade their four seasons for a one-season year as long as their arteries carry enough warming blood out to their fingertips and their veins let them stomp through the snow without agonizing calf cramps. Activity-limiting effects of poor circulation make winter seem more fierce, whether from varicose veins, phlebitis, dizzy spells, cold hands and feet, or blood-lack leg cramps. Home remedies and correctives can hold all of these conditions at bay, though. Several tried-and-true techniques will help you to keep both your veins and your arteries working well and to recognize and combat circulatory conditions which account for more hospital operations and more lost limbs than any other disease in the world. Let's start with the most common, most easily identified conditions, and then move on to the other frequent complaints stemming from diseases of veins or arteries.

HOME MEASURES AGAINST VARICOSE VEINS

Home measures alone may entirely cure small varicose veins. You can control the misery which larger veins cause, slow their growth, and prevent many of their complications with home measures.

How to tell if you have varicose veins. You can check yourself for varicose veins without a doctor's help. Bare your legs and stand perfectly still for about three minutes beforehand. Use a single lamp for a light source. Examine the portion of the leg where the light strikes tangentially, just where the leg's curve makes it fall into shadow. Turn slightly or move the light to bring other areas into vein-revealing focus. Any vein in the lower leg larger than a lead pencil indicates that vein valves have given way. More advanced varicosities show up as winding, enlarged surface veins. Tiny sunbursts of surface veins need not be considered: your doctor can eliminate them with injection treatments if you wish, but they do not cause circulatory problems.

Home measures can stop the formation or growth of varicose veins. You can keep small, beginning varicose veins from growing larger and keep new varicosities from forming by controlling or interrupting leg vein engorgement. Ordinarily, the calf muscles squeeze on the deep leg veins with each leg motion and send a spurt of blood up along the main leg veins. When the muscles relax, the deep veins fill with blood from the surface veins. Valves prevent the blood from backing up into surface veins during muscle contraction, and still allow it to flow freely at other times. These valves look like shirt pockets sewed lengthwise to the inside of the veins. When the blood flows from the surface veins to the deep ones, it goes past each pocket from the closed end. When the blood tries to flow from the deep to the surface veins, it runs into the open end of the pocket-like valve which fills and balloons out into the vein passage. Each valve pocket is barely big enough to stop up the vein at its ordinary size. If you stand or sit still for a long time, the vein may become engorged and stretch until it is too large for its valves to close off. Blood backing up from the deep veins stretches the surface and connecting veins further. This leads both to the unsightly, wormlike surface varicosities, and to breakdown of more and more vein valves.

You can usually stop varicosity formation completely by taking these three steps:

1   Eliminate vein-engorging constrictions and pressures. Free flow of blood from the leg veins to the heart makes valve-impairing engorgement much less likely. The main way to guarantee free flow: Wear loose-fitting clothing that does not bind at the knee or thigh, especially no stockings that have tight elastic bands at the knee.

2. Pump blood out of your leg veins frequently with muscular action during prolonged sitting or standing. From either sitting or standing posture, rock up on your heels, lifting the toes of both feet as high as possible. Return to normal position. Rock up on your toes. Return to normal position. Repeat three times every 20 to 30 minutes.

3. Flush veins thoroughly with the aid of gravity drainage every two hours during prolonged sitting or standing. This exercise is a great refresher, whether you have normal leg veins or varicosities. Take off your shoes. Lie on your back, and bring your legs up until your knees are directly above your head. Stretch your legs and feet straight up, bracing your hips with your hands. (Alternate method: lie with hips on the arm of an overstuffed davenport and with legs stretched straight up.) With feet and ankles entirely relaxed, jiggle the legs with short, rapid to-and-fro motions. The flopping about of the foot milks fatigue-causing wastes out of the muscles and flushes the leg veins thoroughly in about 30 seconds.

HOW TO CONTROL VARICOSE VEIN MISERIES. If you have lead-pencil-size varicosities, they probably cause more fatigue and discomfort than you realize. Varicose veins make your feet and legs tire very quickly, lead to frequent foot and leg cramps, and sometimes impair circulation to the skin of the lower leg so badly that it becomes congested or develops open sores. Varicose veins decrease the effective circulation in the other, deep-lying veins of the leg without in any way replacing it. When the leg musculature squeezes on the deep leg veins, they squirt blood past the ineffective surface vein valves into the stretched, stagnant varicosities instead of toward the heart. When the leg musculature relaxes, blood from the varicose backwash pours back into the deep veins. The muscles and other tissues get only a fraction of the circulation they deserve because the deep vein pumping action is wasted on back-and-forth movement of stagnant blood.

Gravity-aided vein flushing. With mild varicose veins—enlargement, but no tortuosity—gravity-drainage vein flushing usually keeps varicose veins from impairing the circulation in your legs. The communicating veins in such cases are usually not so badly stretched that their valves do not work at all: the valves only fail when the veins become engorged. Frequent vein flushing keeps engorgement from occurring. Follow the gravity-aided vein flushing program described above every two hours throughout the day, and every hour during periods when you are usually standing or sitting still.

Elastic bandages. Elastic bandages keep most varicosities from impairing your circulation. Smooth, steady pressure from the outside keeps surface veins from absorbing the blood that should rush on toward the heart. Get a four-inch elastic bandage (two lengths if any veins above the knee are enlarged). The rubberized bandages give snugger support than plain cotton, although some patients must use plain cotton because rubber irritates their skin. Keep the remaining bandage rolled as you apply each turn, and stretch the bandage about halfway to its maximum length as you wind it on. Apply two anchor turns around the ankle. Carry the bandage down from the front of the ankle for a turn around the foot. Now spiral up the leg, overlapping approximately half the width of the bandage on each turn. If more than one length of bandage is needed to extend above the highest engorged vein, fasten the end of the first bandage with the hooks provided or with safety pins, then start another bandage with one or two turns overlapping the first bandage and spiral on up the leg. When you reach the knee, bandage with the joint partly bent and take two or three Figure-8 turns—one loop below the knee, one above, joining at the back of the joint. Continue your spiral and fasten the bandage top as before.

Long underwear. Many patients (even women) find that the easiest way to keep a bandage in place is to wear long cotton knit underwear underneath it. If you do this, you can draw the bandage somewhat tighter. Be sure that the knit fits snugly enough to be relatively free of wrinkles and folds.

Supphose. Support stockings are not quite as effective as elastic bandages, but are much more convenient and attractive. Some brands, such as Jobst, are made to your exact measurements, which makes them almost the match of an individual bandaging. If your proportions are close to average, less expensive brands work equally well.

Periodic leg exercises. An elastic bandage allows normal muscle movement to push blood along toward the heart. However, it does not increase the efficiency of circulation while you are sitting still or standing. You should get in the habit of pumping the blood out of your leg veins every few minutes when you are standing or sitting still by rocking up on your toes and heels alternately.

Take a few days' home treatment for varicose veins even if you think they aren't hurting you. Leg aching and fatigue from poor venous circulation come on so gradually that victims often do not realize how much trouble their enlarged leg veins are causing. As one of my patients told me:

"Until I got my veins fixed, I thought aching feet and weariness were just part of getting old. When your feet and legs wear out, you feel worn out all over. But it just doesn't happen like that any more. I can keep going all day, and then some!"

Try a full-scale program for vein misery control if you have varicose veins, whether you think they are causing you trouble or not. You might be surprised at how much energy and comfort you can restore. I've seen dozens of patients lose complaints they thought were due to old age through simple vein care.

When your doctor can give worthwhile help for varicose veins. Even in cases formerly ruled as incurable, modern surgical techniques almost always give permanent relief for varicose vein suffering. If any of your lower leg veins is bigger than a lead pencil, you should discuss the problem with your doctor during your next visit.

The presence or imminent danger of open sores is a more pressing reason for getting medical care for varicosities. Open sores usually form on the outer side of the leg just above the ankle. Redness, itching, and scaling or brownish discoloration in this area usually precede ulcer formation by several weeks or months. Any of these signs in combination with moderately severe or severe varicose veins should send you to your doctor in a hurry. With prompt attention, you may save yourself the misery of a months-long smoldering infection.

Although most experts today prefer operation to injection treatment, a permanent cure for varicose veins involves much less disability and discomfort than most people think. One or two days in the hospital and a few more days at home usually solves your vein problem for good. The procedure causes much less pain than any abdominal operation. The biggest barrier is cost, which is usually about the same (for both legs) as for an appendectomy.

HOW TO WARD OFF PHLEBITIS

You can frequently keep raw or clot-plugged veins from troubling you by taking simple measures at home. If phlebitis does strike, you can often avoid serious risks by deciding promptly what is wrong and taking the proper steps.

How to prevent fireman's phlebitis. Most firemen freely admit to poor physical condition. For weeks on end, they sit around the station playing pinochle and leaning on a polishing rag. Then comes a four alarm fire and they run up and down ladders like a bunch of boy scouts in a relay race. No wonder two or three men show up with phlebitis after each major fire! Unaccustomed, prolonged exertion plays havoc with delicate veins. However, our Minnesota hunters and outdoorsmen have found three rules which help them to keep clear of this problem:

1. Train up to heavy exertion. Take a walk each evening in the weeks before hunting season, practice a few minutes every day for a week or two before you try your first 18 holes of golf.

2. Bracket periods of exertion between a good warm-up and a slow tapering of activity. One of my patients always walks several blocks to the tennis courts and back, for instance. He's still good for three sets at age eighty-two.

3. Use elastic bandages or support hose for extra vein support if these steps are impossible.

How to dodge the phlebitis of immobility. The phlebitis of immobility is next in susceptibility to home measures. Whenever you go to bed for several days without getting up or moving around, your circulation becomes quite sluggish. Especially in your older years, the risk that slow-flowing blood will clot in the veins of the legs or pelvis is quite real. You can avoid this hazard by following two rules:

1. Never stay in bed continuously without consulting your physician. Complete bed rest is a very dangerous treatment unless precautions are taken against phlebitis. Even if you're sure you'll soon get well, an illness which keeps you from getting up to eat and to toilet yourself deserves medical care.

2. When you stay in bed with a cold or other minor illness, make it a point to change your position in bed every fifteen minutes while you are awake. Roll on one side, then the other. Prop yourself up on several pillows, then let yourself back down. Exactly the same principle holds when you are under a doctor's care. If your physician doesn't give you specific orders about moving around in bed, be sure to ask him what you should do. Moving in bed is especially important after surgical operation and obstetric delivery, so take special care to keep mobile at such times.

How to interrupt migratory phlebitis. The form of phlebitis next most likely to yield to home measures is clotting of the veins underneath the skin. People who are subject to such attacks get them repeatedly, in different parts of the body. Each vein heals into a firm, non-tender strand in ten days to three weeks.

You can make further attacks of surface vein-clotting much less likely to occur if you discontinue the use of tobacco. Since this condition is sometimes a vanguard of other more serious circulatory problems, this step is well worthwhile. If will power alone won't free you of the smoking habit, try Chapter 17's suggested techniques.

How to ward off infectious phlebitis. The last form of phlebitis which you can avoid through home measures is due to involvement of the vein walls in the spread of infection from a surface sore. The techniques for controlling skin infections which we discussed on page 172 will keep this kind of spread from occurring.

How to spot phlebitis before serious complications occur. Most serious vein clots occur in the deep veins of the lower leg. Every movement of the calf muscles presses on these veins, so you suffer some discomfort on walking and on tipping the foot upward. Pain is never severe, however, and is sometimes barely noticeable. The blocked vein passages lead to slight swelling of the ankle and foot. Some patients have a degree or so of fever.

Phlebitis in surface veins or varicosities makes the vessels firm and tender, usually with some reddening of the skin above them. Your doctor can use medicines to keep the clot from spreading into the deep veins if you call him promptly.

Aspirin. For many years, doctors thought that the stomach bleeding which sometimes follows excessive aspirin use came from irritation of the sensitive lining. Recent studies showed a different and exciting cause. Aspirin, even in moderate doses, stops one of the early stages of blood clotting. What formerly seemed a dangerous side-effect now has become a very important and helpful medicinal action of aspirin. Two tablets twice a day help to ward off and sometimes even cure blood clots in both veins and arteries. This action occurs even when the effect of aspirin on the stomach itself is avoided by taking it after meals or with milk. Regular twice-a-day use of aspirin cures or prevents many forms of phlebitis and often keeps down damage from hardened arteries in the legs or in other parts of the body. I prescribe this dosage for any patient who shows signs of mild or moderate circulatory problems in any vein or artery. Severe circulatory disease calls for more powerful blood thinners, of course, and these require a doctor's close and continued care.

HOW TO CONTROL DIZZY SPELLS

You can sort out several types of dizziness through simple tests and observations. You can get substantial, lasting relief from many of these conditions with little or no expense or discomfort through home care. You can decide promptly which spells call for a doctor's care. Here's a step-by-step program for handling dizzy spells that covers all of these points:

What to do when dizziness strikes. Lie down perfectly flat with your eyes closed and your head stationary. While the dizziness continues, check these points to help guide your management of future attacks:

Do you seem to whirl, or does the room whirl around you?
Do you get worse when you move your head?
Is your breathing deeper or more constrained than usual?
If you can feel your pulse, is it rapid or slow?

After the attack subsides, consider the answers to these four questions and the circumstances in which the dizziness occurred. Try to determine which of these forms of dizziness plagues you, and take appropriate action:

Balance organ dizziness. If the room seems to be whirling around you, your dizziness is probably due to sensitivity of the balance organ inside of your ear or irritation of the nerves connected with that organ. Further confirmatory test: moving your head rapidly from side to side will make you temporarily worse, and sometimes will also make you sick to your stomach. Effective home measures:

1. Nose drops, ¼ per cent neosynephrine or ½ per cent ephedrine in isotonic saline (available in many states without prescription, and perfectly safe for everyone except victims of severe heart disease or high blood pressure). Lie with your head over the side of the bed, lower than the level of your chest, turn your head to one side, and put two drops in the lower of the two nostrils. After 30 seconds, turn your head the other way and put two drops in the other nostril. Repeat every four hours for two days.

2. A low salt diet, which is usually needed for at least six weeks. No salty foods like ham or potato chips, no salt added either in preparation or at table to other foods.

3. Motion sickness pills, either Dramamine or Bonamine, which you can get at any drug store without prescription.

These measures have only about a fifty-fifty chance of bringing the attacks of dizziness under control. If they fail to bring about marked improvement inside two days, you should see your doctor.

Overbreathing-type dizziness. One type of dizziness almost always responds to home measures: overbreathing alkalosis (also known as "hyperventilation"). The attack starts with giddiness and light-headedness, usually accompanied by tingling of the hands, feet, and sometimes the face. In severe cases, muscle spasms make the hands draw up and the toes curl. The initial light-headedness gradually goes on to frank whirling sensations. This series of complaints is actually due to rapid, deep breathing. Such breathing blows off an essential portion of your blood's main acid substance, leaving the body alkalies in full control.

Rebreathing. If you hold the opening of a large plastic bag snugly against your face and breathe in and out of it, overbreathing type dizziness will usually abate. Rebreathe the same air for two or three minutes, even though it seems to be getting stuffy. Empty the bag of old air and start rebreathing again immediately if symptoms are not entirely under control.

Breath holding. You can usually nip attacks in the bud by holding every other breath at the first sign of giddiness or tingling. Continue for six to ten breaths, or until symptoms abate.

How to manage fainting type dizziness. Some dizzy spells are simply a mild form of fainting. Sudden giddiness during an emotional crisis, at the sight of blood, or in the presence of pain is due to emotional reaction in the blood vessels, detouring blood that would otherwise supply the brain through vessels leading to the muscles and abdominal organs. The blood-starved brain seems awhirl. If you lie flat or sit with your knees spread wide apart and put your head far down between them, the attack usually passes off.

Posture change dizziness. When you stand up, the arteries in your legs have to get very much smaller and the arteries in your neck quite a bit bigger. Otherwise, the blood goes to your feet, leaving your brain poorly supplied. Your arteries may not make these adjustments instantly when you sit or stand quickly. You become lightheaded from lack of circulation to the brain. No serious disorder is responsible. The complaints usually disappear if you sit down and put your head between your knees. People who are subject to this complaint should get in the habit of sitting on the side of the bed for a few moments in the morning and getting up deliberately whenever they have been sitting in the same position for a long time.

Carotid sinus dizziness. If dizzy spells on position change develop in later life, especially if the pulse is markedly slowed during each attack, the chances are that sensitivity of the artery-controlling nerve centers in the neck is at fault. These centers are located on the main neck arteries approximately at the level of the top of your voice box. If they become oversensitive, any position change or any slight pressure over the carotid sinus area can throw you into a severe faint.

One of my patients had this type of difficulty. He had attacks almost every Sunday for months. Problem: the high, starched collar which he only wore for church services rubbed the carotid sinus area. Since he's switched to soft-collared sports shirts, he hasn't had a single attack.

If you think carotid sinus sensitivity might be your trouble, test yourself for it in your own home. Lie down, turn your head slightly to the right, and press the ball of your right thumb against the pulsating artery just to the left of your windpipe, opposite the top of the voice box. Roll the thumb around the surrounding area slightly. If dizziness occurs, release the pressure immediately. If the left sinus proves insensitive, wait at least three minutes before testing the right one. Never under any circumstances press on both sinuses at once.

You will probably find that you can control your complaints by wearing soft open collars and avoiding sudden position change even if your carotid sinuses are quite sensitive. If these measures fail, your doctor can arrange to snip the oversensitive nerves. This operation is quite minor and leaves no serious after-effects, but it almost always gives permanent and lifelong cure.

Low blood-sugar dizziness. Giddy spells, dizziness, or actual faints can stem from a low blood-sugar level. Your brain has no reserve supply of fuel, and blanks out when the blood fails to supply its needs. Usually this problem arises when you have skipped breakfast or gone without food for 12 hours or more. Excitement or tension may also play a part. In some susceptible individuals, attacks occur in the rebound phase an hour or two after any heavy carbohydrate meal (such as waffles with syrup). A soft mint, sugar cube, or glass of sweetened orange juice gives almost instant relief. For prevention of further attacks, see the discussion of hypoglycemia in Chapter 2.

Dizziness from medicines. A number of medicines can cause dizziness in people who are unusually subject to their action. Aspirin and the aspirin family, nose drops, nerve quieters, antihistamines, codeine-containing cough syrups, and many other common remedies may be at fault. If dizzy spells develop while you are taking any home remedy, discontinue it for two days to see whether the dizzy spells disappear. If dizzy spells develop while you are taking medically prescribed remedies, telephone your doctor.

When your doctor can give worthwhile help for dizzy spells. You need your doctor's help to discover and treat any possibly serious underlying disorder if your dizzy spells are accompanied by other complaints or alterations in body function. Victims of anemia usually complain of fatigue as well as dizziness. High blood pressure causes headaches, loss of wind, and other difficulties along with dizziness. Heart disease almost always causes pain, weakness, or breathlessness before it causes dizziness. Severe diarrhea or vomiting leads to dizzy spells through upset in body salt and fluid balance. Internal bleeding from an ulcer or other condition may cause dizzy spells along with weakness, black, tar-colored stools, and cold sweats. Your doctor can give you substantial help for each of these conditions.

HOME MEASURES FOR COLD HANDS AND FEET AND FOR BLOOD-LACK LEG CRAMPS

You can take several effective steps to combat sluggish blood flow through your arms and legs. The most common complaint from poor circulation is a cold numbness of the hands and feet. With more severe involvement, patients in the late thirties, forties, and fifties complain mainly of circulation-stopping spasms brought on by cold exposure. Their fingertips turn blue and become very painful whenever their hands become slightly chilled. Older patients are less subject to spasm and more subject to muscle cramps. At first, pain in the calves of the legs occurs only after very prolonged walking or running. As time goes on, the amount of exertion required to bring on an attack steadily decreases, until some victims can only walk half a block or so without pausing to rest. Proper home treatment often boosts circulation enough to vanquish these complaints.

Warm clothing. When your body is trying to conserve body heat, special passages open up between arteries and veins in your hands and feet. This short-circuits blood flow from the surfaces of your fingers and toes and cuts heat loss from your body, but it also makes your hands and feet uncomfortable. To keep your body from taking this step, all you need to do is maintain a higher internal temperature. A sweater, down vest, or "long johns" does more for cold hands and feet than mittens or foot packs, and interferes less with freedom of movement. A fur hat or warm cap is also very helpful—the many blood vessels in your scalp never constrict with cold exposure, so that about 30 percent of heat loss from your body occurs at this site.

Hot towels to the adjacent trunk area. You can increase the circulation to any important body part with heat, but YOU MUST NEVER APPLY HEAT DIRECTLY TO PARTS IN WHICH CIRCULATION IS IMPAIRED. The trick is to warm the trunk area which shares nerves and blood vessels with the affected part instead of warming the part itself. This makes the blood vessels to the affected area open up without increasing the affected tissue's need for oxygen and fuel, as direct hot applications would do. Before age sixty, most circulatory problems have an element of spasm which can be relieved promptly by hot applications to the upper part of the extremity and to the adjoining trunk. Especially if the attack has been aggravated or brought on by exposure to cold, by emotional upset, or by excessive smoking, hot towels to the shoulders and upper arms or to the thighs and hips are worthwhile. Dip the towels in water at 112 degrees, wring partly dry, put them on, and cover with a sheet of plastic or with a dry towel to cut cooling from evaporation.

Warm flannel. After age sixty, gentle, more sustained warmth will gradually bring comfort and improved circulation. Wrap the affected part in warmed flannel or put on long cotton or wool underwear. Use a cushioned heating pad set for low heat across the shoulders or hips. Keep the rest of the body comfortably warm, since heat-induced sweating may make you somewhat subject to chill.

Smoking and circulation. Nicotine increases arterial spasm as long as arteries retain their elasticity. Circulatory difficulties which strike before age sixty, and especially those involving painful blue fingers or abruptly freezing toes, are often greatly improved if you quit smoking. You'll find a helpful home routine to aid you in this difficult task in Chapter 17 of this book.

Aspirin. For prevention of future difficulty, two aspirin tablets twice a day taken after meals or with milk often work wonders. Aspirin works in this situation by preventing blood platelets from clumping together and either obstructing the blood vessels or serving as the starting point for a clot. Once you have evidence of sluggish circulation, take aspirin in twice-a-day dosage continuously. Unless something better comes along, I would recommend that you continue aspirin for life.

How to boost your circulation with home exercises. You can substantially improve the circulation in your legs with Buerger-Allen vascular exercises if you are plagued by coldness, numbness, or cramps. These exercises are very easy to perform right at home. The object is to stretch and stimulate the tiny blood vessels in which the greatest resistance to blood flow occurs by alternately overfilling and draining them. Plan to do Buerger-Allen exercises three times a day for at least three months before you decide how much good they are doing: effects are sometimes slow, but usually occur if you persevere. Here are step-by-step directions:

1. Turn a straight chair over on the lower half of your bed, so that the legs of the chair stick out over the foot of the bed and the chair's back forms an angled platform for your legs when you lie down. Pad the back of the chair with a folded sheet. Lie down on your back with your legs lying along the inclined chair back. Remain in this position for two minutes.

2. Sit up with your feet dangling over the side of the bed. Slowly and deliberately carry out each possible foot and toe motion: turn your toes down, raise them up, turn your feet inward, turn them outward, spread your toes, and close them again. Continue these motions for three minutes.

3. Lie flat in the bed with your feet and legs wrapped in warm blankets. Relax in this position for five minutes.

How Dave Porter improved his waning circulation. Dave Porter's case shows what Buerger-Allen exercises and twice-a-day aspirin can do.

"I've always thought it was better to wear out than to rust out," Dave told me. "But I'll be blamed if I can keep going any longer! When I try to mow the lawn I can put in just about three turns around the yard, then that's it. Leg cramps! Get so I just can't stand up any more."

Dave was sixty-two, but from the knees up he looked and acted like a man in his late forties. Only the arteries in his legs seemed to be markedly hardened, but one look at the dull, mottled skin of his ankles and feet proved that he was only a few months away from a case of gangrene. I recommended exercises and aspirin, but with great fear that they would prove futile.

A year later, Dave Porter marched with his lodge brothers on a two and a half mile parade without a spasm or cramp. Aspirin and Buerger-Allen exercises—exactly the same as the ones you can do at home without a penny in medical expense—had helped him to unclog his blood vessels. He has remained active for several years now without further difficulty.

Further aids to circulation. If home measures fail to restore circulation, your doctor can suggest many other highly effective techniques. You should never settle for a life hedged about with circulatory limitations simply because people have always talked about these things as immutable burdens. Your doctor can arrange diet and medicines. He can help you to rent inexpensive circulation-stimulating equipment which you can use right in your own home. One hopeful fact: I have never seen and never expect to see a person robbed of a limb by gangrene without months and months of warning symptoms. Pale, lifeless color, sometimes with dry flaking of the skin, coldness to the touch and loss of feeling are good reasons to get your doctor's help. Blood-lack calf cramps, cold feet, and mottling are even earlier warning signs. If you remain alert for lack of circulation, you can bring a legion of home measures and medical aid into the battle to prevent gangrene.

16

How to Make Your Heart and Arteries Last Longer

Too many people are afraid of long life. Age means misery and disability to them: steady decline to a pitiful remnant of their former selves. How wrong these pessimists have proved! Science today can promise that if you combat and hold off the heart and artery diseases which are our most deadly plagues, you will not suffer the miseries and disabilities that people have always blamed on old age. You will add *youthful, vigorous* years to your life.

This is no idle dream. Although further discoveries will certainly shed more light, you can already get effective aid from thoroughly known facts in meeting every one of these life and death problems:

How to win speedier, more complete recovery if a heart attack strikes.
How to get extra help from your doctor for heart and artery troubles.
How to cure frightening but innocent chest pains.
How to fend off hardening of the arteries.
How to avoid coronary heart attacks.
How to keep your blood pressure down.

You can apply the main measures in each of these crucial spheres right in your own home. Here are exact directions.

HOW TO WIN SPEEDIER, MORE COMPLETE RECOVERY IF A HEART ATTACK SHOULD STRIKE YOU

Better than four out of five people who suffer a heart attack get back to full-time work and a potentially happy life afterwards. Most of the rest recover well enough to be happy and useful again. If a heart attack strikes you or someone you love, you can do a lot to hold down damage. The outcome of an attack often depends on what is done in the first few minutes,

222

when the doctor hasn't yet arrived. Here's how to handle each of the two main kinds of heart attack when it first strikes:

PAINFUL ATTACKS can best be fought flat, right where they occur. A coronary heart attack strikes with crushing pain in the middle of the chest. The pain may run down the arms or up into the neck. Dizziness and a cold sweat often follow. If you suffer such symptoms, the first thing to do is lie down (even on the floor or ground). Impaired circulation otherwise could diminish blood flow to vital centers such as the brain. Extra warmth also helps the circulation, so you should get someone to cover you with a blanket or coat.

Emergency life support. For several years, I have been debating with myself about the benefits of Emergency Life Support units. These ambulances with special equipment and trained paramedics now service most metropolitan areas and a number of smaller cities and towns. They bring electrocardiograms, oxygen, injectable drugs, and skilled medical advice (via radio communication) to the heart attack victim wherever he might be, usually within two or three minutes after receiving a call. The plusses of such care are obvious: I have seen the special injections and electrical devices used on these units actually start up a man's stopped heart. Another doctor and I had kept the victim's circulation going and breathed air into his lungs, but we would never have saved his life without the Life Support Unit's help. The minusses are more subtle: all that hustle, bustle and excitement certainly pumps adrenalin into the victim's veins, and that's the last thing on earth that he needs.

As the figures accumulate, though, I have finally recognized that the plusses outweigh the minusses by a considerable margin. If an Emergency Life Support unit is available in your community, write the phone number on the cover of your telephone book right now. Give them an immediate call if you think that anyone in your household might be having a heart attack. The hustle, bustle and excitement might be bad, but the treatment is good enough to more than make up for it.

Rest and calm. If you do not have access to Emergency Life Support, the next best thing is still rest and calm. Absolute rest of body, with all the emotional and mental calm he can muster. Except in a fully equipped and staffed unit, a coronary victim shouldn't be moved from the place of their attack for at least one hour, and often not for two hours or more. A doctor should be at the victim's side, of course. The victim needs relief of pain, which only a doctor can bring. But the doctor can come to the victim's side without sacrificing the crucial help of total rest, while a wild ride in an ambulance unequipped to deal with the disturbed heart rhythms and other effects of excitement might do terrible harm.

Here's how Pete Armstrong helped himself through a heart attack: Pete Armstrong woke in the middle of the night, fighting for air against the frightful pressure in his chest. He clutched at the lamp on the bedside table, which crashed to the floor. His wife woke with a start.

"What's wrong?" she said.

Pete only gasped. She reached out to him. Her hand struck the dank coldness of his face.

"My God!" she said, and leaped for the light switch.

"It must be my heart," Pete gasped. "There's a pain in my chest and down my left arm."

"I'll call an ambulance, right away," his wife said.

"No," Pete said, raising his hand. "First get me blankets. I'm supposed to lie quiet, and I'm so cold I'm shivering."

His wife got the extra covers.

"Now call the doctor," Pete said. "But don't just say to come out and hang up. Ask him what we should do now." He closed his eyes and lay quiet. Relaxing in the face of fear and pain was the hardest job he'd ever tackled. He did his best.

"The doctor's coming," his wife said, back at his side. "He says you're doing fine. Just stay relaxed."

That just what Pete did, as best he could. He spent as little effort as possible, physically, mentally, and emotionally. That fact, more than what his doctor did for him, helped him to recover quickly and completely.

SMOTHERING-TYPE HEART ATTACKS. Suppose the heart victim doesn't have chest pain. Instead he wakes up at night choking for breath. Or he finds that he needs to stop after every slight exertion to catch his breath, and finally can't breathe naturally even when he's holding still.

Such smothering spells usually come from heart trouble. However, you can still have long years of fully useful, happy, and contented life when they strike.

A lazy, chair-borne ride. A quick, effortless trip to oxygen and medical aid is the key to prompt cure for smothering-type heart attacks. That's what a heart victim needs, and it's usually easy for him to get it without paying ambulance fees. The sitting posture is better than the lying one, anyway, and it takes less time to load up and leave than to call for help.

How Muriel Johnson pulled herself through a smothering style heart attack. Muriel Johnson shook her head. She just couldn't get her breath. Middle of the night or not, she had to have help. She called her brother.

"What's wrong?" her brother asked when he burst in.

"It's my heart, I believe," Muriel said. "Don't get upset, though: The doctor warned me that this might happen, and told me what to do."

"He'll come right out?"

"No, he'll meet us at the hospital. Call him for me now. Then get some help and carry me down the stairs. I'm supposed to stay right in this straight chair. Tip me back and carry me as far as the car: that's the easiest way on both of us, the doctor says. Then you're to drive me to the hospital, and they'll give me some oxygen."

Muriel stayed calm and relaxed while the men hoisted her down the steps.

"I'll make an apple pie for you when I get back," she said between heaving breaths. "But right now I'm supposed to keep still."

She did a good job of it. Ten days later, she was back to a full program, and able to make that apple pie.

Rescue squad. In most cities, the fastest way to get oxygen for a smothering type heart attack if you can't get to a hospital is through the fire department's rescue squad. Fire department equipment always includes oxygen, and workers are trained in its prompt use. Although some ambulances carry excellent oxygen equipment, others have nothing whatsoever to offer. If the situation seems desperate or your doctor cannot be reached, the rescue squad may be your best bet.

HOW TO HELP YOUR DOCTOR GET THE JUMP ON HEART AND ARTERY TROUBLE

Your doctor can offer help for many heart and artery troubles, but he can't do anything until you decide that something might be wrong and visit him. On the other hand, undue alarm at every twinge of chest pain keeps many people miserable and broke. How can you spot the conditions which your doctor can help without undue alarm or expense?

Heart complaints don't mean heart trouble even half the time. Here's one cheerful fact: if you go to your doctor because you think you might have heart disease, the odds are overwhelming that your heart will be all right! Here's a list of complaints which send patients into a tailspin of worry and concern, when actually they seldom mean heart trouble or any serious bodily disease at all:

Pain under the left nipple or low in the left chest.
Palpitations or pounding of the heart.
A smothering sensation with deep and slow breathing.
Light-headedness with numbness of the hands and feet.

Even real heart failure can be stopped before it starts. Most people think that the heart beats faster and harder when it gets overburdened, and then suddenly quits. They've had plenty of chance to soak up this false and terrifying idea, from the very words ''heart failure'' to well-meant but scare-type propaganda.

Don't let left-overs from such old-fashioned nonsense frighten you! If your heart ever finds itself under strain, it'll give you plenty of warning. You'll have time to get help, and the help you get will stand you in good stead.

Twinges of heart misery give valuable warning. Brief heart discomfort may give enough warning to let your doctor ward off an impending coronary heart attack for you. Such heart misery comes on abruptly. It usually strikes with overload from heavy activity, strong emotion, or extra eating. The pain is in the middle of the chest, and seems to cut off your breath. One patient called it ''a fist shoving into my chest''—not a cramp, a searing pain or knife-like twinges, but a feeling of world-crushing weight. Discomfort may spread up to the neck or down either arm. One tip-off is that the victim instinctively sits or lies down and stays quite still during an attack instead of restlessly rolling or moving about. Don't confuse such pain with mere indigestion. Attacks like this, even though they pass off in a few minutes, mean that a doctor's care can help you a great deal.

Sluggish heart action. Sluggish heart action or leaking valve trouble gives its first warnings through swollen feet and congested lungs. When the heart doesn't pump blood freely from the veins, pressure backs up to the tiniest, least water-tight vessels. The blood juices leak out. When you are up, the weight of the blood makes extra congestion in the feet and ankles. Swelling occurs there. At night, this swelling leaves. With the whole body level, fluid pools in the spongy lungs, which become water-logged and inefficient.

That's the background for the early signs of sluggish heart action, namely:

Evening swelling of the feet and ankles. When you notice this sign, press your finger firmly on the swollen area for ten seconds. If it leaves a definite dent, see your doctor the next day, even though the swelling has disappeared by then.

Too quick loss of wind with exertion. Breathing is rapid and shallow, with the chest partly full all the time. Things you could ordinarily do without trouble, like walking up one flight of stairs or working at a normal rate make you lose your wind.

Loss of wind in the middle of the night. Patients often tell how they get up in the middle of the night because the room seems stuffy. A few minutes' sitting by the open window relieves them. But it isn't really the open window that helps: it's sitting up so that the fluid siphons downhill out of the lungs to other body parts. If such a spell hits you with the rapid, shallow breathing of true heart trouble, prop yourself up on three or four pillows or in an easy chair. If the attack doesn't subside, get help. If it does, go see your doctor in the morning to avoid further difficulty.

Rheumatic fever. Don't you get a wonderful feeling of relief when your doctor tells you that there is no leak in any of your heart valves? You can enjoy that feeling through the years, thanks to a new advance in medicine. Most leaky valves come from rheumatic fever, and rheumatic fever now can be held off by killing the family of germs that triggers each attack.

Penicillin or sulfa. The American Heart Association gives penicillin top billing for rheumatic fever control. One or two tablets a day almost always prevents the heart-crippling form of rheumatism. Sulfa derivatives fill in for patients who can't take penicillin. You should check with your doctor about this technique if you've ever had rheumatic fever, inflammatory rheumatism, or a rheumatic-type heart murmur. Under these conditions, one visit to your doctor and one or two pills a day will practically eliminate your extra risk of valve leakage.

HOME CARE CAN BANISH MANY INNOCENT CHEST PAINS

Proper home measures cure almost all of the pains and twinges in the chest and upper abdomen that cause people concern and discomfort without actually being due to heart or lung disease. Probably the most common such condition is *pinched nerve chest pain*, which causes steady, dull discomfort or sudden twinges along one or more rib segments. This condition usually strikes after you have been sitting in a cramped position for several hours: driving a car, working at a desk with one arm hanging unsupported from your shoulder or the like. The weight of your shoulder and arm pushing down on your ribs lets the muscles between the ribs pinch tender nerves. The pinched nerves make these muscles cramp tight, causing still more damage. The next day you suffer from pain in one side of your chest, most often on the left but sometimes on the right or on both sides. You can get relief from pinched nerve chest pain by this simple exercise.

Chest stretching. Sit sidewise in a straight chair, preferably with a back high enough that its top falls just opposite your nipple, with your left side toward the chair back. If the chair back is too tall, sit on a telephone book or cushion. Let your left arm hang behind the chair so that your ribs are against the chair back. Reach your right arm straight up toward the ceiling. Bend your right elbow and put the fingertips of your right hand on your left ear. Now bend your body across the chair back, tipping your right elbow as far as possible toward the left and stretching it up toward the ceiling. Let the chair back press against your left chest to act as a fulcrum. You should feel your right ribs spreading apart. Stretch the rib muscles in this way for three seconds. Switch to the other side and follow the same procedure. Stretch each side three times. Follow the whole routine three times a day until pain ceases. Ward off further discomfort with stretching exercises once a day thereafter.

Gas pains sometimes strike high enough in the chest to cause considerable confusion, too. The highest portion of your stomach, in which gas frequently accumulates, tents up underneath your diaphragm nearly to nipple level. Gas pains are generally on the left side instead of underneath the breastbone. They do not run down the arm as heart pain often does. Attacks sometimes follow over-eating or unusually rich food. A dose of bicarbonate and a carminative enema (see page 82) often give quick relief.

HOW TO FEND OFF HARDENING OF THE ARTERIES

Free blood flow through supple arteries keeps all your organs supplied with fuel and gives blood clots no harmful place to form. The conditions that cut short the lives of nearly half of all Americans cannot strike. The decline people blame on old age will not visit you: enough moving blood keeps your memory sharp, your skin young, and your muscles strong.

Hardening of the arteries is a controllable disease. Hardening of the arteries comes from a scaly deposit in the wall of the blood vessels which carry blood to the tissues. This scaly deposit is made largely of cholesterol, a substance found in food, and also formed within your body during digestion of the fat that you eat. Hardening chokes off blood flow and makes rough places on which blood can clot. Clogged circulation means decline, which is what people fear about "old age." But the trouble isn't age! Hardening of the arteries is a disease that science can now prevent and even cure.

Why cholesterol forms scales within artery walls. Although nobody can prove exactly what chemical steps take place in depositing cholesterol within the wall of an artery, certain general principles seem established. Cholesterol and its chemical cousins form in vast quantities within your body when you eat certain fats. None of these substances dissolves freely in the blood or tissue fluids. Your body floats them through the circulation on protein rafts—giant molecules with soap-like ability to keep fatty substances suspended in water or blood. As tissue fluids filter through the artery wall to nourish it, some of these protein rafts get stuck. They are small enough to pass through the artery's inner lining, but too large to move all the way through the vessel wall. Chemical processes ultimately break down the trapped protein raft, leaving its cholesterol-molecule passenger stranded within the artery wall. The thickening and abnormal character of the vessel caused by the presence of cholesterol soon makes passage of other protein rafts still more difficult, leading to more and more stranded molecules, like traffic backed up from a single road-blocking stalled car during a Minnesota blizzard.

Attacks on the artery-hardening mechanism. Several links in this disease-forming chain are now being subjected to research attack. New soap-like substances have been found which carry the cholesterol on through artery walls, but unfortunately have proved to have undesirably poisonous qualities. The difference in protein rafts, only a small proportion of which are large enough to get stuck in their passage through the vessels, has been studied very intensely. Several substances have been found that greatly alter the size and shape of these rafts. One such substance is heparin, which unfortunately has profound effect on blood clotting and may lead to deadly hemorrhage unless dosage is rigidly controlled. Another such substance is made by the body in response to heparin and seems safe and effective, but cannot yet be manufactured. Perhaps new discoveries at any time will spell the end of hard arteries' deadly toll and prolong life for half of all Americans. Meanwhile, we can only control this condition by dietary and living methods. These have been conclusively proved to slow or reverse the hardening process, but only when applied day by day over a period of many years.

The fat you eat determines the cholesterol in your blood. Even though you eat considerable cholesterol in such foods as eggs, butter, and cream, dietary cholesterol makes little difference to your blood cholesterol level. The acids and enzymes in your stomach and intestine destroy much of the cholesterol in your food before it even soaks into your system. Cholesterol formed inside your body, from fats which you eat, really constitutes the bulk of the cholesterol in your blood at all times. Unless your body uses fats in an abnormal way, your program for lastingly supple arteries need not include any restriction on cholesterol-containing foods, which are tasty and easily obtained. Only a few people have abnormal cholesterol blood tests and need to follow a strict doctor-prescribed diet.

On the other hand, the amount and type of fat you eat very definitely affects your blood cholesterol content and therefore the rate at which your arteries become hard. Polyunsaturated fats, which tend to be liquid at room temperature, do much less harm than saturated fats, which tend to be solid.

There is no doubt that your arteries will last longer and stay more supple if you eliminate as much saturated fat as you can practically do without, both by substituting liquid for solid fats and by limiting total fat intake.

You can find on any grocer's shelf the foods you need for keeping your arteries much more supple. You would have to give up many good foods if you wanted to go all out for supple arteries. But you can cut hardening of your arteries in half by choosing delicious, satisfying foods from your grocer's shelves. You can do this with no extra food costs at all, because no special foods are required. Just follow these three rules to keep supple, long-lasting arteries and younger tissues through the years:

1. Keep down the amount of harmful fat you eat with your meat. Eat harmless (or possibly helpful) veal, fish, or poultry twice a week. Trim off all visible fat from all types of meat. Avoid fat meats like bacon and fried or panbroiled meat, which has soaked up extra fat during preparation. Choose "economy" or "good" grade beef and pork instead of fatter "choice" or "prime."

2. Use liquid cooking oils in preference to solid shortenings whenever possible. Fat added for seasoning or as an ingredient and fat which soaks up into food during frying make up a large proportion of the fat you eat. Natural vegetable oils are not only harmless to your arteries but also help to cancel out the deleterious action of animal fats. The chemical processes ordinarily used to make such oils into solid shortenings convert them into the type of fat most researchers now feel is most harmful so you should use the oils in their natural, liquid form. Teflon coated pans and spray-on shortenings, such as Pam, help to keep food from sticking with a minimum of cooking fat.

3. Keep the total fuel value of your foods down to the level which will support your body at its ideal weight. The absolute amount of undesirable fat you eat is what counts the most. Even if you follow the above rules, you will get at least 25 to 30 per cent of your calories from fat. (The American average is 42 per cent.) At least half of that fat will be of the undesirable animal or solidified variety. (The American average is 85 per cent.) You can eat enough of such food to sustain you at normal weight without worrying about your arteries. If you eat half again as much, your total intake of undesirable fat is nearly back where it started. A program to cut your weight back to its ideal level and keep it there is often practical (see Chapter 18), while more stringent limitation in proportion and type of fat is absolutely impossible without laboratory-prepared foods. That is why weight control is a key step in gaining full artery-sparing effect.

An artery-preserving diet is tasty, varied, and easy to follow. You can spare your arteries without depriving yourself of the pleasures of a well-set table. For example, look at the slight modifications one of my patients had to make when he took up this program. In the left column is the menu he would have followed ordinarily. Next is his new menu. Last an explanation of the changes involved.

ORDINARY:	ARTERY-SPARING:	CHANGES:
Breakfast:		
Grapefruit	Grapefruit	Omits fatty meat (bacon) and uses vegetable oil instead of animal fat for frying
Fried eggs and bacon	Eggs fried in vegetable oil	
Toast	Toast	
Coffee	Coffee	
Lunch:		
Roast beef sandwich	Chicken sandwich	Substitutes chicken for beef, since he has no strong preference and poultry fat is less harmful than beef fat
Tossed salad with French dressing	Salad (same)	
Apple pie (crust made with solid shortening)	Apple pie (crust made with vegetable oil)	
	Milk	Makes crust with oil
Dinner:		
Panbroiled sirloin steak	Broiled sirloin steak	Steak broiled so that fat drips off instead of soaking back up into the meat
Baked potato	Baked potato	
Peas	Peas	
Lettuce and tomato salad	Lettuce and tomato salad	Peas not seasoned with butter or oleo in the kitchen
Chocolate cake	Chocolate cake	Cake and icing made with vegetable oil instead of solid shortening

If this patient had been a bit overweight, he might have made further changes. Boiled or poached eggs instead of fried, fresh fruit instead of pie, low calorie salad dressing or vinegar, and a low calorie pudding like D-Zerta instead of chocolate cake would knock perhaps six hundred calories off his day's total. After his weight was down, though, he could switch to a program like the one listed, which places very little strain on either the cook or the consumer.

Readers who wish to follow a somewhat more rigid artery-sparing diet because of past difficulty with hardening of the arteries, coronary heart attacks, or stroke, or because of a strong family tendency toward such illnesses, will find helpful directions and recipes in any of the several "heart patient" cookbooks available in any good bookstore.

Even easy artery-sparing diets may soon be unnecessary. If you eat out at restaurants or have poor control of how your food is prepared for other reasons, there's a bright ray on the horizon for you: close chemical cousins of cholesterol, called sitosterols, can be used to block the pathways which artery-clogging substances take into your bloodstream from the intestine. The effect on your body when you take sitosterols as medicine is the same as if you stuck to a very low fat diet, and more—some additional cholesterol may be flushed out of your body. At the moment, this treatment is quite costly. The time may soon come when we can enjoy lots of rich or fried food and supple arteries, too, without prohibitive expense.

HOW TO AVOID CORONARY HEART TROUBLE

When you avoid hardening of the arteries, you'll avoid coronary heart attacks, too. A great many heart attacks are due to stopping up of one of the arteries through which the heart muscle itself gets fuel. A clot is what stops up the artery, but clots only form after hardening has made the vessel narrow and rough-walled. If you follow the dietary measures we've discussed to keep your arteries supple, you'll help your heart dodge most coronary attacks.

Three other measures give you further help:

1. You can open up your coronary arteries with muscular activity. Daily, mild muscular activity opens your coronary arteries. This makes coronary heart attacks less common and less severe. British mailmen, for example, walk several miles each day. They have fewer heart attacks than postal clerks with similar salary and status. The few mail carriers who have heart attacks get much milder ones than the clerks suffer. People who do heavy work have only one-third as many heart attacks as people who do light work according to Drs. Jeremy N. Morriss and Margaret D. Crawford of Britain's Medical Research Council. In this country, nationally known authorities like Dr. Paul D. White have long recommended regular exercise for every reasonably healthy man or woman, regardless of age. All of these top doctors agree that steady activity helps both by opening up existing coronary blood vessels and by making extra detour channels develop, so that the plugged coronary arteries which cause most heart attacks become less likely and less harmful.

Exercise. You can put yourself in the nearly-heart-attack-free class by gradually building up your own activity unless you have severe disease-imposed limitations. This activity ought to be regular and mild. Most people find that walking a mile or two daily, riding a bicycle to and from work, spending an hour in the garden or at the bowling alley, or any of a dozen other interesting, useful pursuits will fill the bill. The important things are these:

1. Pick something you can do daily.
2. Use heavy leg and trunk muscles mainly: then you can exert enough effort to stimulate your heart without tiring yourself out.
3. Have a special activity planned for bad weather, off seasons, and times when your schedule gets crowded.

Why not set up a program right now? Write down what you want to do, including second-bests. Decide right now to bowl twice a week if you can and to take a walk after supper whenever you can't. Or decide to spend an hour in either your garden or your workshop every day. Barring doctor's orders to the contrary, keep up this custom until you're 90 or more.

2. Aspirin. Two aspirin tablets twice a day, after meals or with milk, definitely make coronary clots less likely to form in narrow vessels. Many doctors use a prescription-only chemical cousin of aspirin instead, but the accumulating evidence seems to show that aspirin is just as good.

3. You can develop wholesome outlets for pent-up emotion. You have seen for yourself what strong emotions can do to human blood vessels. The pale face of fear, the flushed face of anger—almost all emotions involve violent and visible shifts in the size of surface blood vessels. Exactly the same changes occur in your inner organs. Different arteries clamp down during some strong emotions, engorge themselves during others. When vital arteries clamp down, blood flow in them slows, especially near the scale-narrowed spots in hardened arteries. If severe slowing occurs throughout your body, your blood pressure soars. If severe slowing strikes in the coronary vessels, a clot may form and cause a heart attack. Likewise with many other parts of the body: stopped blood vessels can cause stroke, sudden blindness, gangrene, and so on.

Such trouble develops mainly when tightness of the arteries continues for hours. Since emotion-induced tightness disappears when you express your feelings, ordinary emotions do no harm. Your blood pressure may soar when you're angry, but it drops quickly when you've said your piece. Only pent-up emotion creates lasting strain. Wholesome outlets for your feelings completely protect your body from most harmful effects of emotion.

What wholesome outlets? Three main ones are worthwhile:

A. Express your feelings freely whenever possible. You need considerable self-control. However, self-release is safe and useful, too. Some matters aggravate you, but aren't big enough to merit self-control. Some differences involve people who love you enough that they'll forgive a minor flare. In such circumstances, why not practice self-release on purpose, as you now practice self-control?

One of my coronary patients seemed quite meek. He never blew his top at anyone. Yet he was always inwardly upset. He boiled for hours after his wife called him "Baldy." He got mad as hops when his teenager took the family car without asking permission.

"Why don't you ever sound off?" I asked. "Tell them how you feel. You'll feel better, and they'll try not to annoy you quite as much."

"Maybe you're right, but I've never said a word before. I don't know how my family will react."

"You'll never know until you try. Just speak up right away whenever you're annoyed, in your own home. That'll be safe enough, I promise."

He tried blowing off steam with his own family. By the end of the month his heart condition was much improved, and so was his disposition.

"I'm doing the same thing at the office now," he told me. "I used to be afraid to say how I feel for fear people wouldn't like it. But they seem to like me better when they know just where they stand."

That's what he liked about his new behavior. But what I liked was something different: the pills he used for heart pain were all still in the bottle. He hadn't needed a single one. If too much self-control keeps you constantly constrained, and if your family's feelings can stand up under a little temporary upheaval, you will probably find similar release worthwhile.

B. Discuss and air your feelings. When you tell someone what has happened to you, you live the events over again in your mind. Can't you use this fact to set your feelings straight? To gain release and sympathy, and perhaps the satisfaction of saying all the things you wish you could have said, but didn't at the time?

One of my patients always used my offices this way, with my wholehearted consent.

"There's no one else I can talk to," he said one day. "My family's wound up in this, and my friends all gossip."

"Tell me about it," I said.

"It's my wife. She's always siding with my daughter Rose. The girl's getting sort of wild. Last night, I told her she'd have to stay home for a week, she'd been late so often. But my wife just told her to go on out with her boyfriend.''

"I guess that made you mad, all right.''

"Mad? I just couldn't open my mouth for fear of what I'd say. The others went on out to do the dishes—this happened right at supper—and I picked up the paper, but I couldn't read. I was in a perfect stew. I should have stormed right in there and told them a thing or two, that's what I should have done.''

Does this conversation sound futile to you? It wasn't really. In the end, my patient calmed down and made up his mind to make the best of his home situation. He felt much better for going over his upheaval with me, even though it didn't really change things.

Perhaps you'll find some problems you can discuss with your close friends, your family, or your religious adviser. Perhaps you'll find it helpful to write letters, even if you never send them through the mails. Air your feelings! It's a real help, both to your mind and your body.

C. You can take out strong feeling on a substitute. One way to rid your body of pent-up feeling is to take it out on someone or something else. This certainly is bad at times: I don't advise anyone to beat his wife if he's had trouble with his boss, or kick his horse when his in-laws make him mad. But there are some substitutes that work perfectly well without making trouble or stirring later pangs of conscience. You can chop logs. You can hit golf balls. You can shoot rabbits. Such violent actions help to blow off steam without troubling your conscience or disturbing your life with your neighbors.

Do you need such release for yourself? Here's a brief self-quiz that will help you to decide. Answer these questions yes or no:

1. When someone has said something unpleasant or unfair, do you often think of a good retort when it's too late?
2. Do you feel abused sometimes?
3. Are you extremely proud of your self-control?
4. Are you frequently frustrated?
5. Do you feel wound up and tense for several hours after a disagreement?
6. Have you had high blood pressure or spells of heart pain?

If you answered "yes" to two or more questions, you definitely need a way of blowing off steam regularly. One "yes" means you could use such release at times, but needn't work it into your daily program. In either case, pick an appealing method from the list below, or choose something similar that suits your own needs. All these things let you attack something

physically, or give you the feeling of being in on such an effort. They're all
entirely proper.

Safe Ways to Vent Your Spleen

Participation Sports:	Spectator Sports:
Golf	Watching football
Bowling	Watching wrestling
Darts	Watching hockey
Hunting	Watching boxing
Archery	
Tennis	

Hobbies and Crafts:	Household Tasks:
Whittling	Carpentry
Woodworking	Scrubbing floors
Coppercraft or metalcraft	Hand laundry
Sewing (in part)	Chopping wood
Leather tooling	Parts of cookery, such as
Gardening	pounding meats, mix-
	ing batters, chopping
	nuts

You can meet some resentments specifically. If there's one obvious
thorn in your side, you can take even more specific steps to make it
painless. Take the case of a union chief and how he handled this problem,
for instance:

"You say I should let loose," he told me. "But I sit at the bargaining
table with those slick-smiling goons, and I've got to smile, too. They're
cutting the heart out of my plans, and they hate my guts. But I've got to
work with them. It's my job to coop up my feelings."

"At the same time, yes," I said. "But what about later?"

"When? After I quit this job?"

"No, each day. I'm going to have you paste their pictures on the wall
down in your basement. I want you to throw darts at those guys. Score it
however you please—ten points for an eye, five for a nose and two for an
ear. Play with someone or all by yourself. But put in fifteen minutes at it
every night."

Sound foolish? Maybe so. But it worked. My patient felt great relief. If
someone constantly pushes you around and you can't talk back to him try
one of these prescriptions: Throw darts at his picture. Paint his likeness on
your chopping block. Picture him in your mind's eye as you take aim at a
target with rifle, shotgun or bow. Think of his nice round head when you

wallop a golf ball. You'll feel the pent-up anger flow from you as you carry out these plans.

HOW TO KEEP YOUR BLOOD PRESSURE DOWN

What makes blood pressure high? The arteries through which the blood flows become narrow, then the heart has to push extra hard to force blood through. The narrowed or tense arteries come first. The pounding, over-active heart comes later, if at all.

The measures we've discussed for keeping arteries supple help to hold your blood pressure down. Wholesome outlets for emotions also help: they relax all the arteries in your whole body and lower your blood pressure. These measures are extremely important, but there are also several specific ways to fight off high blood pressure.

Hold your blood pressure down by dodging excess salt. African tribes without ready access to salt don't suffer the scourge of high blood pressure. People who never salt their food or salt only to taste are less likely to have high blood pressure than those who salt their food without tasting it first. Although this has never been proved to be a cause and effect relationship, it seems reasonable to skip excess salt.

You can hold your blood pressure down through self-assertion. Like strong feelings, strong urges need outlets. When your just impulses are curbed, your blood pressure soars. Most experts say four out of every five cases of high blood pressure stem from such stresses rather than age, physical disease or strain. It's a dangerous tendency you can spot in yourself, as a frequently occurring frustrated, overtight, hurt feeling.

What can you do instead of fume inwardly? You can get in the habit of asserting yourself. Be decisive, definite, and prompt in every issue that is really up to you. That's how my patient, Jim Meadows, straightened himself out.

"People walk all over me," Jim said on his first visit. "My wife, my kids—everybody."

A three-point program changed all that:

First, Jim trained himself to make decisions promptly in areas where no one would argue. He made up his mind right away about what to wear, what to eat, and what to do.

Second, he learned to express himself promptly and definitely. He got rid of such phrases as "I think I'll have thus-and-so" and "Maybe such-and-such would be all right for me." Instead, he said "I'll take thus-and-so" or "Give me some of that, please."

Third, he said what he thought about contestable issues *before* the other fellow spoke up or took action. He trained himself to speak up quickly, without worrying about what the other fellow might think, whenever he was responsible for ultimate decisions.

At the end of a month, Jim told me:

"I'm on the right track."

"Why, what's happened?" I asked.

"My wife *asked* me what I wanted to do last weekend instead of just making plans. First time since we've been married."

"Did you have your suggestions ready?"

"Well, not this time. But next time I will."

I'm sure he did. Jim didn't remake himself entirely—nobody ever does, or ever has to—but he made himself a power to be considered in his own home. In the process, he lost his feeling of pent-up containment and relieved his extra proneness to high blood pressure.

You may help your high blood pressure by getting reassurance. The actual facts about blood pressure aren't as bad as most people think. If your blood pressure has sometimes tested high, you can take comfort from these facts:

> *Moments of emotional upset won't cause a stroke no matter how high your blood pressure goes.* Tests of the strength of brain arteries show that the highest pressures researchers could produce, more than five times the peak to which blood pressure rises in the worst cases of hypertension, do not blow out normal arteries. So forget the frightening notion that a stroke will punish you for slight anger if your blood pressure's up.
>
> *High blood pressure does not move inevitably toward higher pressure, heart failure or stroke, and death.* Most patients with blood-pressure readings above normal either revert to normal at later rechecks or keep a safe, if slightly elevated, pressure for life.
>
> *You're not better or worse according to your exact blood pressure reading at the moment.* It's the condition of your kidneys, blood vessels, and heart that really determines whether high blood pressure will cause you trouble. If your doctor can reassure you on these points, that means a lot more than the level of your blood pressure itself.

Doctoring for blood pressure. In recent years, a number of new medicines have become available for high blood pressure. One or another combination almost always can get the numbers right without substantial side effects. I never start a patient on these medications unless the lower of the two numbers is high on every visit for two or three weeks, but in that instance proper medication can take a lot of strain off of your system.

17

How to Meet and Conquer
Tumor Threats

"Cancer Death Rate Cut in Half!"

That's a headline everyone on earth would love to read. Yet it could be written today as far as you and your family are concerned. If you put present day knowledge of cancer to work, you can cut cancer's probable toll at least in half. You can prevent many cancers entirely. You can get complete, lifelong cure twice as often as the present average if cancer strikes. Even if the disease gets too far along for complete cure, you can often win a years-long reprieve while research bores closer to the ultimate cancer cure.

You can avoid many cancers altogether. The most hopeful word in the cancer field is this: as many as nine out of ten cancers of certain types, including several of the most common, can be avoided entirely! That doesn't mean merely that a painful, expensive operation can keep the victims out of the grave. It means that nine out of ten who would have had these forms of cancer can keep themselves from ever having an unhealthy day or needing a single treatment.

How can this be? Because science has proved that one big factor in starting many cancers is irritation. There are other factors, too—family tendencies, hormones, cosmic rays, and probably a dozen more that haven't been discovered yet—but the straw that breaks the camel's back is irritation. Avoid cancer-spurring irritation and you'll very probably avoid many varieties of cancer.

Irritation spurs cancerous growth. Bits of tissue are growing continually in your body. But they grow only to replace worn-out or injured bits nearby. The difference between normal tissue, simple tumors or growths, and cancerous growths is simply a matter of degree. All tissue grows. Tumor tissue grows more than it should, and presses on surrounding parts. Cancer tissue grows so violently that it can eat into normal tissue as well as press upon it.

Irritation definitely affects cellular growth. Anything which continually injures tiny bits of tissue so that they have to be replaced spurs more growth than would otherwise be needed. This increase in the rate of tissue growth sometimes spurs the exaggerated growth of cancer.

HOME MEASURES TO EASE
CANCER-SPURRING IRRITATIONS

If you set out to dodge cancer-spurring irritation, a great deal of what you can do requires no medical aid or expense whatever. Here are three big steps:

1. Shield yourself from cancer-causing ultraviolet rays. Farmers and sailors get eight times as many cancers of the skin as indoor workers. The reason: excess sun exposure, with damaging amounts of ultraviolet light. Only the areas of skin exposed over a period of many years become increasingly cancer-bearing—the face, neck, and hands.

You can dodge excess ultraviolet rays without staying indoors or otherwise inconveniencing yourself. Don't worry about brief in-and-out sun exposure. If you will be in the sun continuously for an hour or more, a broad-brimmed hat helps protect your face. A bit of unmedicated yellow petroleum jelly (Vaseline) will protect the backs of your hands or other heavily exposed areas for six to eight hours. A good suntan oil or cream will screen out most ultraviolet light, too. A preparation called "Sundown" blocks almost all ultraviolet, if you need total protection.

2. You can protect your lungs against dangerous fumes and irritants. Scientists have actually found cancer causing irritants in the exhaust fumes of automobiles and trucks. The dangerous fumes are heavier than air. In heavy traffic, you should let fresh air into your car through the windows instead of using bumper-level ventilating ducts. You should also keep your car's exhaust system in good repair so you won't breathe in lung irritants from your own engine.

What about tobacco? Years ago, I used to shrug my shoulders at the quit-smoking crusades. My own consumption was over two packs of cigarettes a day. Then the facts began to pile up incontrovertibly.

What facts?

First, cancer of the lung was proved much more common in heavy smokers. Men who smoked as much as I were 52 times as likely to get cancer of the lung as nonsmokers. Even lighter smokers had a substantial extra tumor risk—pack-a-day men ran 22 times the nonsmoker rate, and half-a-pack-or-less men ran 11 times the non-smoker rate. Counting only the squamous cell cancers, the type tobacco-tar irritation seems to produce, the effect was even greater.

Second, cancer of the lung is a very common killer, especially among men.

Third, heavy cigarette smoking increases the chance of getting all kinds of cancer by two and a half times. It isn't just cancer of the lung—some still-unknown factor connects heavy cigarette smoking with cancer of the stomach, the bowel, the blood, and so forth.

Fourth, cancer-causing irritants have actually been found in cigarette-smoke residues. Animals get cancer after applications of certain concentrated cigarette-smoke tars.

Fifth, studies proved that the lung-lining cells reveal progressively more growth and more precancerous change the longer you smoke. A good lung pathologist can classify how close your lungs have moved to the cancer bearing state, and this judgment coincides closely with your past cigarette smoking habits.

Sixth, no known means of protection removes the risks from continued smoking. Filter tips, denicotined tobacco and so on have not been proved to help. Switching to cigars cuts risk appreciably, but doesn't eliminate it entirely.

Seventh, less cancer isn't the only health benefit to be gained by discontinuing use of tobacco. Smokers of any type have more heart attacks and blood vessel disorders. Smoking hasn't been proved responsible, but if even half the heavy smoker's extra heart and blood vessel troubles are due to the tobacco itself, conquering the habit will add years to his life. Emphysema and several other lung conditions also punish many smokers for too many "puffs."

When I added up the totals in my own case, I found that smoking was slated to cost me at least ten years of life span. I figured it was worth a little discomfort to gain that much time on earth. So I quit cigarettes.

HOW TO QUIT SMOKING

You might get enough satisfaction from tobacco to make it worth the years it costs you. You might want to switch to cigars or a pipe. But if you want to quit smoking, there is one way to make it easier on yourself.

Smokers have a different breathing rhythm than nonsmokers. A nonsmoker breathes constantly at a rate and depth that keeps his body supplied with oxygen and free of certain wastes. The smoker breathes slightly more heavily while smoking and for a few minutes thereafter, then gradually breathes less deeply and less rapidly. Soon he becomes uncomfortable and feels the need of a cigarette. But is it really the tobacco, or the extra blood-purification which will come with smoke-spurred breathing which he craves? An article in *The Journal of the American Medical Association* suggested the latter. As the article suggests, I've had my patients take breathing exercises, then quit smoking while continuing the breathing program. Most of them find that they cut tobacco craving substantially in this way.

What kind of breathing exercises? Left hand on the hip, right hand on the tummy, stand erect. Breathe in through your nose at first without raising your chest. Only after the lung is as full of air as you can get it by moving the diaphragm, which pushes the tummy out under your hand, should the chest begin to rise. Fill the lungs completely, then breathe out slowly through your mouth. Do this ten times, and repeat the whole procedure three times a day. After three weeks, quit smoking but continue the exercises for at least three months. If tobacco craving strikes, take time out for extra breathing exercise. Use any other helpful measures you've found, like gum-chewing or eating extra crackers, along with the breathing method.

Breathing exercises really work. All but one of the patients who have reported back to me are enthusiastic about this program. Here's the most extreme case:

J.G. smiled ruefully when I told him he ought to quit smoking.

"Every doctor I've seen since I got my ulcer has said that," he said. "Believe me, I've tried! Like they say, 'Anybody can quit smoking: I've done it a hundred times.' "

"Let's try it once more," I said. "This time maybe we can make it stick."

J.G. listened with interest while I explained the breathing exercise method. Six months later, he was back for another checkup on his stomach.

"I'm off the weed at last," he told me. "That breathing business really works!"

If J.G. couldn't quit when ulcer pains punished every forbidden puff, I doubt if he ever could have made it without breathing exercises. With their help, he managed to quit at last.

3. You can avoid cancer-spurring irritation by cleansing intimate body parts. Men in the waterless deserts of the world, where bathing is seldom possible, have to choose between circumcision and a high rate of sex organ cancer. A cheesy oil forms under the normal foreskin. If it is left there, it causes irritation. Over the years, this increases the chance of cancer tremendously.

Proper cleansing lets you avoid this tumor risk easily without circumcision. Every uncircumcised man and boy should strip back the foreskin at least once a week during a bath and wash thoroughly, then replace the foreskin in its normal position.

If you're a woman, it's harder to prove that you'll benefit from special cleansing methods of the sex organs. Thorough bathing of the outer portions of the female organ is probably wise at least twice weekly. Douching and other more complex methods have never been proved to ward off cancer.

HOW TO HELP YOUR DOCTOR TO FIGHT CANCER-SPURRING IRRITATION

Your doctor can cure cancer-spurring states at the mouth of the womb. At Memorial Hospital, over a thousand women reported twice a year for ten years to have cancer checkups for their pelvic organs. Two cancers were found, both in an early, readily cured state. But the amazing thing was that there were only two: considering the age of the women studied, doctors had expected at least twenty malignant growths. Why hadn't the other eighteen occurred?

Going back over the records, they found that many of the women had been treated for infection at the mouth of the womb. This infection was of a type that starts by itself, without being spread by sex contact or dirtiness. Treatment for it is painless and cheap, but apparently keeps nine out of ten cancers from ever getting a start.

If you're a woman you can avoid nearly one-sixth of your whole cancer problem by stopping any cancer-spurring irritation at the mouth of your womb. Your doctor's number one job in cancer control is to check the mouth of your womb at least once a year and treat any infection he finds lingering there.

Your dentist can help you dodge cancer. Another important form of cancer-spurring irritation involves the tissue inside your mouth. These cells are often spurred into dangerous types of growth by the rubbing of your cheek or tongue against a harsh place on a tooth or the pressure of a poorly fitted denture or bridge. You get used to these things so that you hardly notice them. But you can easily steer away from big cancer risks by clearing up such states. A trip to your dentist whenever you notice irritating roughness or denture misfits will pay off in banished cancer risks, with the extra comfort a pure gift.

HOW TO IDENTIFY AND RID YOURSELF OF
INNOCENT GROWTHS AND CANCER VANGUARDS

When benign growths or cancer vanguards strike, you can often take curative action for yourself. In other cases, you can assure yourself a quick, inexpensive, and more comfortable doctor-managed cure by spotting the problem and getting help promptly. Consider first the frequently self-cured, benign conditions:

Warts. If you have had a succession of ordinary or plantar warts or have suffered along with medically diagnosed warts because of lack of money or time to have them removed, home techniques may well be the answer.

Dichloracetic acid. Carefully apply a thick layer of petroleum jelly all around the wart so that every bit of normal skin is protected. Dip the tip of a toothpick in dichloracetic acid, obtainable at your drugstore without a prescription. Apply it carefully to the surface of the wart. Use just enough acid to moisten the wart surface. Let it soak in for one minute, then blot once with cotton to absorb excess acid. Clean off the jelly and cover with a small bandage. Repeat the application at three day intervals, trimming or scraping off dead-white destroyed tissue if necessary, until the entire wart and its roots have been destroyed.

Ganglion. A ganglion is a bulge in the lubricated sheath around your tendons. The most common variety occurs on the back of your wrist, and pops up as a prominent, smooth bulge whenever you bend the wrist down sharply. Sometimes the wrist is a bit sore and weak, too.

How to pop a ganglion. The old fashioned cure for ganglions was a wallop with the family Bible, which scattered the fluid from them through the wrist tissues quite thoroughly. Unfortunately, people who use this method sometimes break their wrists if they wallop too hard. A much safer method that works equally well on a thin-walled ganglion is to press down on the top of the knuckles with the heel of your other hand and bend the wrist sharply, then pinch the ganglion very firmly and steadily between thumb and forefinger. Sometimes you cannot make enough pressure yourself to burst the bubble, but one of your relatives can break the bulge between the pulps of his two thumbs.

A ganglion treated in this way may come back, but surgery is no more difficult than it would have been if you had never tried for a home cure.

Skin tags. Many people have tags which hang like tiny punching bags from their normal skin. Such tags have smooth surfaces and normal skin texture. Skin tags are harmless, but sometimes are so located that they frequently become irritated by the pressure of clothing. Your doctor can spark these off almost painlessly with an electric needle, to cure them. If you would rather go through a little discomfort than part with a surgeon's fee, though, one home technique is usually safe.

Ligature removal. If you tie a string tightly around the base of a skin tag, lack of blood will make it wither and die in a matter of seven to ten days. The string must be tight enough to stop up the arteries as well as the veins: otherwise the tag becomes extra swollen and sore. The best way to tighten the string is by winding the ends around your little fingers, making your hands into fists, and pressing your knuckles together like rockers. In this way, you will not rip the tag loose if the string happens to break while you are tightening it.

YOU CAN SPOT MANY CANCER VANGUARDS FOR YOURSELF

Three of the main types of cancer vanguards lie right on the surface of the body, where you can easily spot them for yourself. These conditions are not cancers. However, they are disturbances in cellular growth or stability which frequently allow cancer to start. Your doctor can remove or cure each of these conditions without risk or major expense, and usually without hospitalization or lost working time. Once a month, undress in a well-lit room and look for these signs:

1. Heaped-up skin cells. Some heaped-up skin cells form little horns, curving up to a noticeable point. Others are pearly-gray, dull, dry spots. The most common ones are brownish, rough-edged spots. Whenever any of these types appear, get your doctor to take care of them. If you get many small spots, a freezing spray and quick scrape can make short, painless work of a dozen or more at a visit. If you get a few deeper spots, the electric needle or X-ray will cure them. Many of these respond to Flouroplex, a cream which features a drug originally developed for internal use to fight cancer. This cream is available by prescription only.

Rancher's skin. If you have thin skin, a pink-cheeked, dry complexion, and spend a lot of time in the wind and rain, you are especially likely to get heaped-up skin cells. Cut down the number of spots by washing your face and neck every day and rubbing-in lanolin skin cream. Talk to your doctor about using Flouroplex, which not only heals small lesions, but also reveals the presence of previously unsuspected ones by making them turn red.

2. White patches. Leather-like whitish patches on the lip, mouth, tongue, or female organ are also vanguards of cancer. These white patches most often come where there is some irritation from rough teeth, from a quid of chewing tobacco, or from a stream of hot pipe smoke. Whether you can see any reason for them or not, they are cancer vanguards and deserve a doctor's care.

3. Moles. Most moles are harmless. The few that might be dangerous are these:

1. Moles which you scrape when you shave.
2. Moles on your ankles or feet.
3. Moles which become irritated from the rubbing of clothing or underclothing.
4. Moles which change in size, shape, or color.

How Jim Moore got himself cured before cancer got a start. "I've got this scaly patch on my forehead," Jim told his doctor. "What is it?"

The spot was brownish, rougher than the skin around it, with craggy edges. It felt dry and harsh.

"It's from heaped up skin cells," the doctor said. "It's not a cancer. But if you leave it alone, there's a good chance it'll turn to cancer some day."

"Then I need an operation?"

"Not much of one. We'll inject something to keep it from hurting and burn off the spot with an electric needle. In about three weeks, the scab will drop off and you'll be well."

Ten minutes later, Jim Moore left the office. He was a few dollars poorer than when he went in, but had otherwise suffered no pain. Still, he'd rid himself of a real cancer threat.

HOW YOUR DOCTOR CAN HELP YOU FIND AND REMOVE TUMOR THREATS

Your doctor can find some cancer vanguards which you'd never see. Your doctor can get a good look at parts of your body which you can never see. He knows exactly what to look for. And he can find some cancer vanguards that aren't at the body surface, like growths in the ovaries, inside the bladder or in the large bowel. Whenever you see your doctor for other illness, why not ask him to look you over thoroughly for cancer vanguards, too?

Your doctor can cure many cancers completely. If cancer should strike in spite of everything you do to prevent it, your doctor still has better than a fifty-fifty chance of curing it for you completely. But he can do nothing toward your cure until you take the first step by visiting his office.

When you make your monthly check for cancer vanguards, go through this checklist, too. None of the signs we'll list means that you absolutely have cancer. They only mean that you *might* have a tumor which deserves prompt care. You can double your chance of cure if cancer should strike by seeing your doctor whenever these signs cause suspicion:

1. A sore or spot that does not heal. People often first notice a growth when they bump against it or scrape it. A true cut or scrape should get well within three weeks. After that time, check with your doctor to see whether a tumor might be present.

Most of the time, a true tumor appears as a scab or bump. The scab may fall off or the center of the bump turn angry after a few days or weeks. The spot then looks like a tiny molehill completely surrounding a reddish dent. It usually isn't very sore or tender. Watch for such marks especially on the face, the back of the hands, the lip, tongue and mouth. See your doctor whenever one shows up: if it proves to be cancer, you'll have a better than 95 per cent chance of cure with prompt care.

2. A lump, bunch, or bulge. Take time out right now to find out how your skin and surface parts look and feel. There's probably some knobbiness about your finger joints. There may be clumps of birdshot-sized lumpiness in your breasts. Otherwise, your body should be smooth, and the two sides should more or less match.

When a growth forms on or near the surface of your body, you will be able either to see or to feel it. Skin growths look like tiny raised spots or scabs at first. They feel quite firm. Growths under the skin may show as bumps, but are easier to feel than to see. Growths far beneath the skin may show as a general bulging in the area above them, mainly notable when you compare the two sides. Strip completely in a well-lit room once a month to search for tumors. A shaving mirror with one side curved for extra magnification will help. Feel for lumps, too: you may find some with your fingers which you would miss with your eyes.

Breast examination. If you're a woman, you should check your breasts for lumps with special care. As long as menstrual periods continue, the best time of the month is immediately after bleeding stops. That's when normal gland tissue in the breast is softest and least likely to cause false alarms. After periods cease, make a point of feeling your breasts the first day of every month. Lie on your back with a small pillow or folded blanket under your right shoulder blade and with your right arm curled above your head. Lay your left hand on your right breast with the fingers close together and straight. Use the palm surface of the fingers instead of the tips, and feel by rubbing your hand in a gentle circle. You will catch any lumps against the smooth, solid backing of ribs and muscles. Cover each quarter of the breast in this way—upper outer, upper inner, lower inner, and lower outer. Then bring your right arm down from above your head to your side and repeat, being especially careful to cover the tag of breast tissue that reaches up toward the armpit. Change position and examine the other breast in the same way.

If you're like most women, you'll find two or three areas which don't feel quite right. There will be no real lump, but a sort of inner coarseness. This is normal breast tissue. After an interval, you will get to know how your breast should feel. After that, you'll spot a new lump or thickening with ease. And if you do spot one you'll have better than three out of four chances of lifelong cure, even if it proves to be the worst possible kind of growth, as long as you see your doctor promptly.

Mary Rowen found a lump and lived. Mrs. Rowen sat on the very edge of her chair in my consulting room.

"I'd like you to check my breast, doctor," she said tensely.

Two days later, the lump Mary Rowen had found was in a laboratory bottle and Mary herself was getting well. She's stayed well for many years since, despite the fact that the lump was a cancer. She will stay well the rest of her life, thanks to the one minute a month she spent searching her breasts with her fingers.

3. Unusual bleeding. Here's where human nature does us a bad turn. Things seem to be back to normal in a few minutes after hemorrhage. The natural thing to do is wait to see whether it happens again. The trouble is that bleeding which is due to early, curable cancer may not happen again for weeks or months. Most growths which cause bleeding offer an excellent chance for cure, but each week of waiting wastes part of that possibility. It's smart to watch for these particular forms of bleeding, and see your doctor the first time they show up:

    1. Blood mixed with your urine.

    2. Bloody bowel movement.

    3. Black, tar-colored, soft, and bulky bowel movement, which may mean blood is being poured into the upper intestine and digested into tarry matter.

    4. Bleeding, even involving only a few spots of blood, between menstrual periods or after the menopause. If such bleeding occurs after sexual relations, don't ignore it on that account—that's when first bleeding occurs in many tumors.

    5. Bloody or rusty looking material coughed up from the lungs, or severe, unexplained nosebleeds.

4. Unusual flux or discharge. A watery flow of matter from the female organs which makes the area itch or burn is sometimes due to a serious growth. There are also less serious causes, but this sign always calls for a doctor's examination.

5. Lasting stomach trouble. If you have stomach distress or difficulty swallowing several times a week for three weeks, it's time to talk to your doctor.

6. Change in your bowel habits. Nobody can tell how often you ought to empty your bowels. I've had normal patients who had a movement once in five days, and others who went three times a day or more. But whatever is right for you now ought to be right for you next month, too. If your bowels get suddenly tight or get very loose one week and very tight the next, if you get the feeling that you ought to go but find it impossible to get rid of anything but a little gas, or if you frequently pass little pencil-sized stools, see your doctor.

7. Change in your voice or altered cough. Hoarseness should clear up after two weeks or less. If it lasts longer, get medical attention. You'll win a cure about nine times in ten by prompt care, even if it's the worst thing it could be.

Cough is another matter. Almost everybody coughs up a little loose phlegm once in a while. You probably have to watch for change in your cough, not a brand-new cough. What kind of change? New brassiness, increased depth, accompanying chest pain, foul-smelling or bloody phlegm—any major change should have attention. Again, the odds are that an innocent cause will be found and quickly cured. But if something serious is present, you'll gain by prompt attention.

18

How To Relieve Weight-Related Strains on Your System

This book has often told you that such-and-such a problem would be relieved if you could shed some weight. In particular, weight loss helps almost any disorder of weight-bearing joints—feet, ankles, knees, hips or back. It eases the burdens on your heart and circulation. It takes the pressure off a hiatus hernia and thus relieves some digestive misery. It often relieves skin problems in areas of friction like the groin and the area under a heavy woman's breast. Weight loss often lowers blood pressure enough to let you avoid medical treatment.

Perhaps we should also think of overweight itself as an "ailment." Extremely heavy people certainly suffer higher mortality from heart disease and undergo substantial extra risks when they have any kind of operation. However, those extra pounds are part of *you*, and it is hard for you to think of them as a "disease." I've seen hundreds of patients through the years who couldn't get steamed up about weight loss until *after* they had heart trouble or some other serious weight-related disease. They can stick to a diet when they're fighting a recognized disorder, but simply can't mount an all-out attack on their own poundage before it gets them into trouble.

WHAT TO DO WHEN WEIGHT LOSS IS URGENT

When you need to lose weight in a hurry, a rigid diet like the one outlined in Box One page 257 works best. Your tendency to gain weight in the past almost certainly shows that your usual eating patterns supply more fuel than your body burns. That pattern will assert itself to some degree whenever you *make decisions* about what you eat—even decisions such as how much butter to put on the bread or how large a serving is "enough." The program in Box One leaves absolutely no decisions to be made. If you follow it exactly, you will lose weight.

How much you lose depends on how much energy your body uses up each day. A number of factors enter into energy consumption, including physical activity, exposure to cold air, thyroid function and so forth. One or two pounds a week is the usual minimum, with some patients doing substantially better.

The pattern of weight loss depends on your body's mechanism for calling forth fat from storage. Most people lose five pounds or so quickly, then hit a plateau and lose very little for a week or so. Weight loss then continues in a stepwise pattern—abrupt loss followed by frustratingly long intervals with no progress. A few people "plateau" first: they can follow the most rigid diet for a week or more (sometimes even as much as three weeks) yet lose hardly an ounce. If your body reacts this way, you can take heart from changes in your body contours. Your clothes will get looser, your waist and hips will shrink, and those changes in measurements show that the process of weight loss has actually started, even if it hasn't shown up on the scale. As to which measurements will change first, all I can tell you is that the pounds that went on first usually come off last. Frustrating as it seems, there is no way to get weight off a certain area, such as your hips or lower abdomen, until that particular "storage tank" for fat comes to the top of your body's list.

How Sven Olson knocked off 18 pounds. Sven Olson used the program in Box One to good purpose a year or so ago. Sven had checked his blood pressure on one of those coin-operated machines and got a reading of 148/96 (against a normal of 140/90 or below). That's about where his pressure stood when he visited my office, too, and that raised the question of whether or not he should take medicine.

"Ten or fifteen years ago," I told him. "I wouldn't have even considered giving you any pills for a pressure like that. But two things have happened in the meantime. First, we've gotten a number of medications which can bring your pressure down to normal safely and without side effects—not like the old ones which used to make you drowsy or bring on dizzy spells whenever you stood up suddenly. And second, long-term follow-up on patients with borderline pressures have showed a distinctly increased chance of having a coronary or a stroke within ten years. These studies also proved that you could get rid of all these risks if you got the pressure under control."

"You mean I might have to take some medicine? Gee, I don't like that. Never take any pills unless I absolutely have to—not even aspirin."

"And that's a good idea, if you can accomplish the same purpose any other way. As a matter of fact, there's a good chance that you can. If you'll lose ten or twenty of those extra pounds and take some kind of mild exercise—walking or swimming or riding a bicycle, for instance—your pressure might well come down."

Sven glanced wryly at his own bulging middle.

"I've put on fifteen pounds since I turned the heavy farm work over to my sons. Guess it has crept up on me," he said. "Why don't you give me a diet I can follow and I'll set up an exercycle in front of my TV and grind away for half an hour while I watch the news."

That's exactly what he did, and three months later his weight had dropped from 212 to 194—and his pressure was back in the normal range at 132/86. So far he's managed to keep the extra pounds off, and those blood pressure pills are still in the bottle.

What to do if you need long-term help with your weight control.
Although crash diets can get ten to twenty pounds off faster than any other means, they aren't much help with a lifelong problem. Nobody counts calories (or carbohydrates) for life. So if you need a long-term program, it has to work without arithmetic. The changes in your lifestyle have to be simple and acceptable. Actually, you can get just as much food satisfaction from well-designed reduction meals as from spaghetti and french fries. And if you put the right things on the table you can eat pretty much without constraint. But if your natural appetite makes you eat more fuel than your body burns—and otherwise you wouldn't be heavy—you need to make lifelong changes in your life style to have permanent effect on your weight.

The mental and emotional side of weight control. Some years ago, I cared for a man who had attempted suicide. When I asked him what made him want to end his life, he blamed his diabetes.

"It's always there," he said. "Every meal with your family, every party, every friendly invitation—the red flag waves in front of my face fifty times a day. I can't eat like other folks, I can't drink like other folks, I can't *BE* like other folks. And it just gets to be too much."

To some extent, a weight control program involves this same variety of strain. Your natural eating patterns have made you heavy, and if you eat what you want instead of what you know you should, the weight is bound to come back. So a really workable weight control program involves just as much loss of freedom and just as much interference with your life style as a rigid diabetic diet. And that loss of freedom stirs exactly the same emotional response as loss of health or loss of a dear one. First you deny the facts—it can't really be true, you say, that I can never "do my own thing" again. Then you get angry—why *me?* Why do I have to be different? Then anger turns inward and you feel depressed. Only when you've fought through all these phases can you start to think through what freedoms and capacities you have left, what new freedoms and capacities you may have gained, and what kind of life you can put together within the new set of rules. Even then, you have one more stage to go through. You have to become comfortable with the new order—to absorb the new patterns and feel that they are really *YOU*.

Unless weight control is very important to you (which it should be if it's going to help with life-threatening or disabling disorders), it's very easy to falter along the way. Especially when you get into depression, you feel so miserable, and you *know* that the misery will go away if you simply fall off the wagon. There's no conscious thought involved—you don't say to yourself: "It isn't worth it. I'd rather be fat than depressed,"—but at some level of your mind you know that the lost feeling, the being at sea in an unfamiliar, involuntarily changed lifestyle, will go away if you just dig into a heap of mashed potatoes or a hot fudge sundae. All I can tell you is that this misery will end if you persevere, and that knowing there's a delightful valley on the other side of the mountain can often sustain you through the battle. And it is a battle. Fighting to change your natural inclinations in anything as central as your patterns of food and drink calls for compound gumption. The words "Will Power," with their implication that anyone with any guts would handle the situation with ease, should be stricken from the English languge, at least where they apply to weight. Anyone who has had the problem knows that the pressures he or she feels toward food and drink go far beyond what the "eat anything and stay slim" people ever experience, and that his difficulty in coping with this force stems from its magnitude, not from any deficiency in him.

HOW TO SOLVE YOUR WEIGHT PROBLEM
WITH FITTING SUBSTITUTIONS

Once you face the fact that you need permanent changes in your life style to make weight control work, how do you find a new pattern that will meet your needs and satisfy your urges just as well as the old one?

The answer is SUBSTITUTION. You can control your weight for life yet really give up very little satisfaction or pleasure if you make a series of reasonably even trades.

Substitute protein and fiber for starch and fat. Pure proteins virtually self-destruct. Your body uses as much energy digesting them as it derives from them. Pure fiber passes through your system without ever soaking in. So fish and chicken breasts, which are almost pure protein, and many vegetables and fruits which are 95 percent fiber provide a great deal of food satisfaction at almost no weight-increasing cost. The foods in Box Two, pages 258–259, are all "weight reduction foods" in the sense that you can eat as much of them as you want without doing harm to your weight program. And if you eat them *instead* of your usual menus, you will have given up hardly any food-derived pleasure, but you'll have made huge strides toward getting and staying slim.

Substitute heightened flavor and better seasoning for richness. Of course, even these foods can become weight control horrors if you douse them in butter or coat them with bread crumbs and fry them in deep fat. But there are other ways to make things taste good—in fact to make them taste even better, once you get used to the idea. Several of my patients have told me that they didn't know how good fruit could taste until they followed my suggestions concerning proper ripening, that they really love vegetables now that they've learned to keep the flavor in by steaming and heighten it with herbs, and that they wouldn't think of going back to the deep fat fryer once they've found out the right way to broil. Here are some specifics:

Melon, peaches, pears, plums and so forth all arrive at the store half green, because they bruise easily in shipment when truly ripe. So buy them when they're green and let them ripen. Get a rack or loosely woven basket which allows air to circulate around the fruit, and which has enough area that the fruit can be spread out in one layer instead of piled up. Turn the fruit every day or two, putting the greener side down. (This holds for tomatoes also, which ripen much more evenly if the juices are draining toward, rather than away from, the dry hard parts.) Test for ripeness by color and smell instead of by punching them to test for softness, which will bruise the fruit and mar its taste. With some melons and fruits it is worthwhile to check for ripeness by cutting a small plug with an apple corer. If the fruit is not ripe when tested, the cut-out "circle" of skin or hull can be replaced for a day or two.

Get a steaming rack for vegetables and be sure you never immerse them in water again during the cooking process. Season from above with salt, pepper and herbs such as sweet basil, thyme, marjoram and rosemary. Cook until barely done, not mushy.

Preheat your broiler and start meat quite close, so that its surface sears to seal in juices. As soon as the surface is grayed and sealed, drop the meat to a greater distance from the broiler. Repeat this process on the other side. With thick cuts, sear both sides quickly before lowering the pan and turn one more time to finish cooking the meat through. Season with salt and pepper, garlic (powder, salt or juice), onion salt or marinade rather than with butters or oils. Most fish cuts are so favorable for weight control that you can afford to coat them with lemon butter or the like during broiling without harming their nutrient proportions.

Substitute eye appeal for volume. The word "appetizing" makes you think that the more attractive a certain dish is the more you will eat. But both the dictionary and common sense throw you off the track here: the better food looks the *less* of it you ordinarily eat. I've tried numerous experiments on this point, comparing cheese served in chunks with the same cheese in dainty squares on the tip of fancy toothpicks, comparing balls of watermelon served in a sherbet dish with slices piled on a plate, comparing tuna salad served on a garnished bed with the same salad served out of a central bowl. In every case people eat less when the food looks especially attractive.

The reason is that you become satisfied when the total "pleasure points" in a meal or refreshment reaches a certain point. And eye appeal gives pleasure. So an attractively presented dish meets part of your "satisfaction quotient" before you even take the first bite. Probably the best way to take advantage of this is to put a little extra work into making all the food look good, and some special effort into making your own plateful look good. Some of my patients have lost substantial amounts and kept the weight off for years just by switching to "plate service" and providing suitable garnishes. If you serve yourself in the kitchen or from a sideboard, starting with a plate that already has an attractive garnish (like half a peach on a bed of lettuce or orange sections in a rosette around a dab of cottage cheese), you'll take much smaller servings and have much less inclination toward seconds than if you put everything on the table in serving dishes and help yourself in globs.

Substitute solids for liquids. When you have a tendency toward overweight, it seems as if anything in liquid form just sloshes down into the corners and never fills up your stomach. That goes for milk, orange juice and gravy as well as for beer, wine and booze. Eat an orange and you'll eat less for the rest of the meal. Drink orange juice and you'll eat as much as if you hadn't had anything. Likewise for yogurt or cottage cheese—the same calories you would take in a glass of milk *replace* that extra sandwich instead of sliding down along with it. And gravy or thickened soups can have as much flour as two slices of bread without giving you the feeling of having eaten a thing.

Substitute something—almost anything—for your particular Weight Waterloos. Everyone has Weight Waterloos—high calorie foods that you eat in larger-than-needed quantities. Maybe it's nuts or ice cream or snack foods like popcorn and potato chips. Almost everybody knows his own. If you pick the two things you know do the most harm to your weight program and find a truly acceptable substitute for them, you'll do your weight program a world of good. And the substitute doesn't have to be celery sticks or raw carrots. You're much better off with ten olives than with a bowl of peanuts, or with a banana rather than a dish of ice cream or half a jar of marinated herring instead of a bag of potato chips. These things aren't particularly "low cal," but if you wind up with 100 calories worth of any of them to replace the 500 or 600 calories in the thing they've replaced, you've done yourself a lot of good.

Finally, substitute some low-cal drink for beer or booze. Alcholic beverages blow any weight control program out of the water, both because of the tremendous amounts of fuel they contain and because of their effect on your ability to adhere to the rest of the program. Perhaps a little white wine or an occasional highball can slip through without wrecking the whole shebang, but even these put a substantial dent in your program. If you don't like diet pop or are afraid of artificial sweeteners, try carbonated water with a little lemon, lime, or cranberry juice added. Or try plain ice water—it's amazing how good the old God-given things taste, considering that you never see an ad for them on your TV.

WEIGHT CONTROL SUMMARY

If you need to lose ten or twenty pounds in a hurry, try the program outlined in Box One. A rigid, inflexible diet of this sort works well for almost everyone because it relieves you of all food-related decisions. Just follow it exactly and don't be discouraged if the weight comes off in spurts instead of steadily. Plateaus are a normal part of the weight loss pattern, and may occur early as well as late.

For long-term control, you need lifelong changes in your lifestyle. The six substitution principles set forth in this chapter give you guidelines for developing an eating pattern that you can live with and enjoy while the pounds melt away—and stay off for good.

BOX ONE

QUICK WEIGHT LOSS DIET

Eat only the exact foods and quantities listed. Avoid any other foods or beverages whatever, except unlimited ice and water.

Breakfasts:

½ grapefruit or 1 orange (sectioned) or 2 water-pack figs or plums.
1 egg, boiled or poached
1 piece of dry toast/
Black coffee or tea

Lunches:

Cottage cheese with fruit—Monday with half water-pack pear, Tuesday half water-pack peach, Wednesday 1 slice water-pack pineapple, Thursday mixed with natural (no sugar added) applesauce and seasoned with cinnamon, Friday with 2 tablespoonfuls of water-pack fruit salad, Saturday mixed with fresh blueberries and Sunday with whatever leftovers from the above appeal to you most. Cottage cheese should be 2 percent or low fat, small curd variety.

Dinners:

Monday: 1 polish sausage, sauerkraut, 1 small boiled potato, 1 pear.
Tuesday: Broiled salmon, green beans, 2 tablesponfuls cooked rice, 1 apple.
Wednesday: 1 broiled cube steak, cauliflower, 1 small boiled potato, 1 peach.
Thursday: Broiled filet of haddock, broccoli, 2 tablespoonfuls cooked rice, 6
          Bing cherries.
Friday: ⅓ lb. Salisbury steak (with chopped onion if desired), stewed tomatoes,
          ½ acorn squash, 8 fresh strawberries.
Saturday: 1 broiled veal chop, asparagus, 1 small boiled potato, ½ cantaloupe.
Sunday: ½ broiled chicken, brussel sprouts, 2 tablespoonfuls cooked rice, 10
          fresh raspberries.

BOX TWO

FOODS TO CHOOSE FOR LONG-RANGE WEIGHT CONTROL

Meats: Unlimited quantities of:

Chicken, turkey, pheasant, duck (all without skin). Trout, bass, whitefish, haddock, cod, shrimp, scallops, oysters (all broiled or with breading discarded).

1 normal restaurant serving (broiled, roasted, or boiled with fat trimmed off) of:

Beefsteak, veal chops or cutlet, pork chops or cutlets, ham, corned beef (round, not brisket), leg of lamb, or lamb chops.

Vegetables: *Unlimited quantities of:*

Asparagus	Cucumber	Spinach
Bean sprouts	Dill pickle	Squash, summer
Beet greens	Endive	Tomatoes
Broccoli	Lettuce	Tomato juice
Cabbage	Mushrooms	Turnip greens
Cabbage, Chinese	Mustard greens	Watercress
Cauliflower	Peppers, green	
Celery Chard, Swiss	Radishes	
Cress, Garden	Sauerkraut	

1 normal restaurant serving of:

Beans, string	Eggplant	Peppers, red
Beets	Kale	Pumpkin
Brussels sprouts	Kohlrabi	Rutabagas
Carrots	Leeks	Squash, winter
Chives	Okra	Turnips
Collards	Onions	
Dandelion greens	Parsley	

Fresh fruits:

Apricots	Honeydew melon	Tangarines
Blackberries	Lemons	Cantaloupe
Cranberries	Limes	Rhubarb
Currants	Oranges	Strawberries
Gooseberries	Papayas	Watermelon
Grapefruit	Peaches	
Ground cherries	Plums	
Guava	Raspberries, black & red	

BOX TWO (cont.)

Juice packed or water-packed fruits

Apricots	Cherries, white	Strawberries
Cherries, red	Pineapple	Applesauce
Fruit cocktail	Blackberries	Blueberries
Grapefruit	Loganberries	Figs
Peaches	Raspberries, black & red	Grapes
Pears	Rhubarb	Plums

Avoid fruits packed in either heavy or light syrup.

Cheese, dairy and eggs:

Edam, Gouda, Provolone, Cottage cheese
Yogurt
Eggs, boiled or poached.

Miscellaneous:

Mushrooms, cocktail onions, green olives (not stuffed), marinated herring, club soda with added lime or lemon juice, and dill pickles generally do less harm to your weight program than the things they replace. Artificial coffee whiteners are better than cream for weight control.

Index

Abdominal exercises, 22
Abdominal massage for constipation, 62
Abscessed teeth, 137, 139
Abused feeling, 230–234
Aches, 23
    liniment for, 52
Acne, 166–168, 170–171
Acnomel, 171
Actifed, 107
Activities, 151, 251–252
Adhesive taping, 30–31
    for blisters, 29
    joint strains, 177
Aging, 145–150
Air, dry, 121, 152
Air conditioner, 130
Air pressure changes, 147
Alcoholic beverages, 35, 120, 256
Allergy, 124–131
    food, 39–46, 70
    skin, 157–161
    tests, 40–42
Aluminum hydroxide, 77–78
Ambulance, 223
Ammonia, 168
Amphogel, 77–78
Anabile, 82
Anacin, 135
Anemia, 202–203, 205, 218
Anger, venting, 235–237, 252
Animals and allergy, 131
Ankles, 133, 179
Antacids, 71, 77, 153
Antibiotics, 109, 155
Antihistamines, 107, 126, 128–129
Antiseptics, 185–186
    eye ointment, 142
Anusol, 85, 90
Apnea, sleep, 195–196
Appendicitis, 70–71
Arch strain, 29, 178
Arches, aching, 29–32
Arm pain, 24–25, 52–54, 57, 218–220

Armpits, 185
Arteries, hardening, 140, 147, 228–237
Artery-preserving diet, 230–232
Arthritis, 47–57
Ascorbic acid, 113
Aspirin use, 48
    arthritis, 48, 51, 52, 57
    backaches, 20, 184
    blood clots, 215
    childrens dosage, 111
    circulation, 148, 219–220, 233
    colds, 110, 119
    headaches, 133–136
    muscle aches, 23, 48
    sinus, 124
    toothache, 137
Asthma, 39, 129–131
Athlete's foot, 164–165
Attack, heart, 222–225, 241
Aveeno, 158
Bacitracin, 142, 172–173
Back problems, 19–22, 175, 182–184
Baker, 53–54
Baking soda, 68, 71, 93
Balance organ dizziness, 215–216
Bandages:
    cuts, 186
    joints, 56, 182
    pressure, 56, 181, 186, 211
    sprains, 175–176
Baseball fingers, 179
Baths:
    for aches, 23
    cold friction, 199
    contrast, 27, 29, 57, 180
    paraffin, 51–52
    sheet bath, 201
    sitz baths, 85, 90, 102
    skin healing, 158, 167
    for tension, 197
Bed, for backaches, 20, 183
Bed blocks, 153
Bedbugs, 167–168